C000292433

Mastering Your Crown

A Guide to Transforming Anxiety, Fear, Loss and Grief in Times of Crisis

Emma Gholamhossein

EGholamhossein

Mastering Me Publishing

DEDICATION

To all those who suffer and are brave enough to face their pain.
To all those who have loved and lost and continue to love.

SEE ME

You may see me smile but you don't know my sadness,
You may see me talk but you don't know my thoughts,
You may see me active but you don't know my efforts,
You may see me laugh but you don't know my tears,
You may see my achievements but you don't know my fears,
You may see me happy but you don't know my pain,
You may see me love but you don't know my grief,
You may see me and judge but you don't know my truth.

—Emma Gholamhossein, April 2017

ACKNOWLEDGEMENTS

I would like to thank my parents for their unconditional love and unwavering support. Mum and Dad, it is because of you I believed I could always be whoever I wanted to be. Because of the love and stability you have provided, I have been able to dedicate my life to 'Mastering Me'.

Thank you to my husband, my one true love, for finding me in this life and all the sacrifices you have made that allow us to be together. Eshgham Joonam.

Thank you Mavis Camm, my Soul Sister, and Jackie Bowen for inspiring me with your spiritual work. A special thanks to Robert Light, my true Reiki Sensei, who pushed me to master my abilities and energy.

Thank you to all the astrologers who I listened to and learnt from... Zoe Hind, Merlin Wizard, Cassandra Eve, Alison Chester Lambert, and finally Marcia Wade, the wisest Oracle to the Cosmos.

I would have failed on my writing path without the help and support from: Louise Adams for inviting me to a Writers' Workshop, The Wild Writing Tribe, The Star Sistar Circle, Nicola Bolt, my Soul Sisters Ceryl Bateman and Lynne Jones. I am eternally grateful to you all.

Thank you to all my clients for trusting me and allowing me to share your journey.
I honour and thank all my Reiki students for allowing me to become 'the teacher' but also 'the student' through learning with you and from you too.

Thank you to Cath Wright-Jones for my beautiful logo, to Rhiannon for my Rhi-Flex, to Raegan and Stacey for your earth and water, and to my 'Wet and Wild' besties Helene, Jackie and Lisa T for all your support and giggles. Lastly, thank you to my ever-growing spiritual team.

Sparkly love to you all,
Emma x

CONTENTS

Part 2 – TRANSFORMING LOSS AND GRIEF

Part 3 – MASTERING YOUR CROWN

CHAPTER 1

Introduction

The whole premise of this book is based on the principle of 'basic is best'. I was initially unsure whether it would even be possible to convey all my experiences and insights in such a way, but my intuition and guides assured me that the information and guidance contained within this book was to be clear, simplified and concise. 'That is what humanity needs right now, at this time of great unfolding and transformation, the global deconstruction of an age,' said my spirit guide. Although most of us mere mortals would simply see it as a time of crisis and uncertainty. 'The world's gone mad,' I so often hear. So with that in mind, given that such a mass of conflicting and overwhelming information (some accurate, some not so) has already bombarded our somewhat fragile and overworked minds, I aim to cut through the noise, the confusion, and assist you through this traumatic time and help you regain some sense of balance.

The outbreak of the coronavirus has catapulted the modern free world into turmoil, seeming to turn it upside down. There is much fear, anxiety, panic, anger, confusion, loss and grief being felt by many. When our very existence is endangered and way of life threatened, just know that it is completely normal to feel such wide-ranging emotions. Know that it's OK to not feel OK. Everyone reacts differently in a crisis and to loss, depending greatly on your levels of wounding, unprocessed trauma, mental conditioning, upbringing, belief systems and mental and physical health. But with a little assistance, you can learn how to respond consciously and not just react in a somewhat unconscious and programmed manner.

Whether you believe coronavirus was manmade or natural, leaked from a lab purposefully or by accident, worthy of the status 'pandemic' or not, is irrelevant. Nothing can change the past, and nothing can bring back the thousands of people who have lost their lives. The coronavirus has brought a real threat to life, just like the many other viruses and diseases that could be argued pose a greater threat. However, we are not as informed about those, they are not in our conscious awareness, so we don't fear them as much.

A certain amount of fear is good; it helps keep us safe and mindful. Fear is what alerts us to the threat of harm and danger. However, prolonged fear and anxiety is detrimental to the mind, body and emotions.

Equally, loss and grief are other naturally occurring human emotions that, if not processed properly, can have detrimental effects on our mental, emotional, physical, spiritual, behavioural and social well-being. Many are grieving the death of a loved one, but many more are grieving how life once was. We know the world and our lives have changed, but because we can't see what the new, transformed way of being will look like long-term, we cling to the old in fear. We are in a strange in-between phase of one world dying and another world coming into form.

Throughout the ages, humanity has seen and overcome many disasters, from geophysical tragedies such as earthquakes and tsunamis to hydrological disasters such as avalanches and floods. The Black Death, another biological disaster, killed over 50 million people in the 14th century, and we (especially Europeans) are the living descendants of the survivors. So when the current coronavirus pandemic becomes a part of our history, which it will, how you responded to it and the challenges it brought will be your legacy. You have the opportunity to experience post-traumatic growth, whereby you have a positive psychological change following this crisis. You can learn to create love not fear, togetherness not separation, to thrive and not simply survive. Whether you're experiencing anxiety, grief or maybe both, I aim to bring you some resolution.

I hope to bring you a sense of calm where you become centred and more at peace in the current storm and somewhat chaotic, uncertain world we now find ourselves in. Finding stability from within is what is needed now. At the eye of a storm is complete stillness; I aim to lead you there.

Mastering Your Crown will help you reclaim your power and authority, bringing balance to your mind, body, emotions and subtle energy. According to the Oxford English Dictionary, the word 'corona' comes from the Latin word for 'wreath' or 'crown', and it is my hope that this book will assist you in regaining your sovereignty... the authority to govern yourself. However, the guidance contained within this book is not only limited to the coronavirus crisis, although that was the catalyst for me writing this book. Life will always bring ups and downs for us all, and the steps and exercises contained within are timeless and can be used to transform anxiety, fear, loss and grief at any time.

CHAPTER 2

My Journey

My name is Emma Gholamhossein (pronounced goal-am-hossein... much easier than it looks) and I transformed my own anxiety, fear, loss and grief after a personal crisis in 2016. Following guidance given to me by my spirit guides and using my own extensive knowledge and experience of balancing mind, body and subtle energy, I was able to heal myself.

I experienced anxiety and panic attacks when I was in my late teens, and since that time have been on a quest of self-discovery and self-healing. My 'Mastering Me' journey began by learning about the physical body through my Sports Science Coaching Degree and job as a Fitness and Exercise Instructor. Due to my anxiety, I was soon led to heal my mind through self-taught meditation and practices such as yoga, tai chi and reiki (a Japanese natural healing system). This organically led me to begin healing my spirit/soul—which can sound a little flaky, I know. Hearing this can create a certain judgment, perception and misunderstanding if you are not into that sort of thing. So being the equally scientific, grounded and level-headed person I am, I will refer to that part of my being simply as my consciousness. Once I graduated, I began learning about the diseased body and became a Health and Exercise Specialist working with special populations and those with various medical conditions. Eventually I moved on to teach health, fitness and sport at a university for fifteen years and gained a Master's Degree in Physical Activity and Health.

Alongside my teaching career, I continued to develop my healing practices privately, and in 2010 I had what is known as a spiritual awakening, I discovered that everything is energy (has a vibration and frequency) and began to see and hear into other dimensions of existence. As an academic and unreligious person, it took me a long time to be comfortable speaking about my ability to communicate with spirits and other energetic beings. I like proof, I like quantitative data, and I have this need to understand how something works—plus, how would I be taken seriously as an academic if I told people I spoke to angels? So I just kept it quiet to avoid being branded 'coo-coo' or 'out there'. I had spent over ten years focused on managing my mind, committed to my personal meditation practice, which was a way to ensure my anxiety and panic attacks didn't reoccur, my method of self-care I guess. What I didn't realise was, during that time, the hundreds of hours spent in meditation developed my consciousness and ability to hold and work with my body's chi (life force energy). Although the spirit world was another dimension I was now able to access, I unconsciously feared this, so I guess I turned a blind eye and made the decision to keep working with reiki, angels and crystals instead. I began treating others and quickly realised that I could see the subtle energy of other living people. Their aura (energy field), their chakras (energy centres) and meridians (energy lines). I could see inside people, sometimes even hearing their thoughts. I was so in awe of my experiences, like a child wearing 3D glasses for the first time, and through self-exploration, I waded through, trying to make sense of it all.

Although I had practised meditation for over ten years, it had always been alone in the privacy of my own home, a means to manage my busy mind. But in 2014, I began attending a group that practised journeying meditation and, much to my surprise, instantly began experiencing past-life memories and visions. Like an eager puppy on an exciting adventure, these sessions opened up another world for me, and it was through these guided meditations that I came to meet my spirit guide, Lone-Wolf, who—just to confuse matters—I came to discover had been my father in a past life. For a period of over two years, my visions helped me learn a great deal about this past life, including how my true love had been a man

I could not be with. It was not our destiny to be together, at least not in that lifetime. When I met my now-husband for the first time at the age of thirty-five, although he was nine years younger than I and from a completely different culture and country, it was an instant attraction and love at first sight. Only it wasn't the first time we had known each other; we were simply remembering our connection. It was a love so powerful that it brought us back together in this life, and within seven months we were engaged and married in a further three. Hossein, my husband, is my Twin Flame, which is a very special and spiritual connection between two people. Two flames from the same spark of consciousness expressed in polarity (opposites). Our meeting and merging was magnetic, intense like a fire had been lit in a part of my being I didn't know existed. It was overwhelming too, because it further expanded my consciousness, triggering even more latent abilities within that I didn't know I had or how to control. My psychic visions, insights into the universe and memory of past lives further increased but started to infiltrate my normal day-to-day life, something I had, until then, always managed to keep separate and contained to meditation practice.

At about the same time, my Nanny Cath passed away and her consciousness came to me just before, which I found confusing and very overwhelming. Although at this point I considered myself a healer, psychic and empath, I wasn't yet willing to accept that I was a spirit medium, a mystic and death doula... a person who can assist souls to pass over. Needless to say, my anxiety and panic attacks increased further, and with them came very negative and fearful thoughts. Losing my Nan opened up a very deep wound, a tsunami of grief that I had left unprocessed, unknowingly of course, not just from this lifetime but from countless past lives, including one that I was yet to be shown. This energy expansion and second, even bigger, spiritual awakening came at a price however, and one night in September 2016, a scary and malevolent being spoke to me... 'You are having a Dark Night of the Soul and no one can help you now.' If I had to pathologise my symptoms, the trauma I experienced that one night triggered Post-Traumatic Stress Disorder (PTSD) and psychosis where I became agoraphobic for several months after. Like myself back then, you may be unfamiliar with the phrase Dark Night of the Soul, which correctly refers to a mystic who has a total collapse in their physical reality and experiences a complete ego death. However if you Google it now, a whole host of inaccurate information has erupted on the internet over the past few years that confuses such a spiritual event with depression and other normal tribulations that life can bring. A Dark Night of the Soul for most doesn't occur as a singular spiritual event involving clarity of past lives as it did for me. It is part of a much larger and longer process of awakening caused by a letting go of your perceived sense of self, triggered by crisis, loss and hardship as you journey through life. Some people can experience several very dark periods of prolonged pain and suffering, physically, mentally, emotionally and spiritually, which contribute towards a person's soul growth and evolution but don't necessarily mean they will go on to become a mystic experiencing a Dark Night of the Soul.

I was very lost, confused and felt very alone because I didn't fully understand what was happening to me at the time. A few years earlier, I hadn't even believed in past lives. So as you can imagine, the whole concept made me feel uneasy and it was a lot to process. But it was this one event that led me to put all of my expertise, knowledge, abilities and faith to the test. I spent the next year learning to master my anxiety, raging panic attacks and episodes of derealisation and depersonalisation, which led me to develop a method called the '8 Step Sequence' that unlocked and eased my body and mind from its fear-frozen state.

Then I spent a further four years working through the copious amounts of unprocessed grief I didn't know I harboured within, easing my emotional turmoil and soul trauma through a process I was guided to use, which I simply call 'Letting Go'. Before I experienced PTSD, I wrongly thought it could only be caused by physical trauma such as war or an accident, and before I started processing my grief, I wrongly thought that could only be caused by the physical death of a loved one. While the passing of my Nan was the trigger to my anxiety and panic attacks, there was so much more to my PTSD and grief than I first thought. I started to question the very nature of my own existence, contemplating the meaning of life, my own mortality and fearing the unknown. I came to realise this was a form of 'Death Anxiety', something many are now facing. It was highly perplexing, because although I could see and talk to angels, even speak to spirits who had departed our physical world, still a part of me couldn't fathom or understand it on a mental level. I just couldn't accept death. I mean, I knew my Nan was fine, I felt closer to her now she was in spirit than when she was here physically, yet that was too much for my human self to comprehend. Physically she was gone, gone in a flash, so still I had to grieve her departure, but I didn't know how to, and I was in deep conflict with myself because what my soul and heart knew and what my head believed were at odds. During this time I saw into invisible worlds, worlds that most can't even begin to imagine. I learnt I was a mystic, seer and shaman. But my biggest challenge came from understanding that the dark being who ridiculed and taunted me, the dark being who I feared so much, was actually me, a part of myself. A part of my psyche/soul from a past life that I had rejected and abandoned, for the crimes she had committed and the pain too great to bear. That was when I came to learn of yet another past life I had lived, that of a High Priestess in North America, whose unprocessed trauma kept my soul in this life fragmented. Such fractured parts create your shadow-self, a term originally conceived by psychologist and psychiatrist Carl Jung in the 20th century, a term that describes all the parts of your being that you loathe and detest, every part you have disowned, repressed and rejected. All the parts you can't face, don't want to face or admit are within you. All the atrocities and cruelties that your soul has ever been part of exist there in your shadow.

During this time, I refused to take any medication because I was too scared. Scared of losing any last little bit of sanity I felt I had left, plus I feared the medical doctors would have locked me up if I had explained of the voices I could hear, the dead people I could see and the flashbacks of that evil spirit... who turned out to be a part of me! At best, they might have medicated me into further confusion and numbness, challenging me with even more weird symptoms to contend with. I think my medical records actually state I had social anxiety, but I know that's not the case. Maybe I did have a chemical imbalance in my brain, maybe I didn't. I just know that initially, when I probably needed it the most, I was too stuck in fear and too scared to take medication. Then as I mentally became stronger, I made the conscious choice not to take it because I realised that my sensitivity is part of who I am. I felt that medication may have suppressed my abilities, which would have meant never truly finding myself; it would have also meant never discovering and developing the 8 Step Sequence or writing this book. Just to clarify, I hadn't been using narcotics or any medicinal drugs, in fact, I never have used them and wasn't about to start either, but with the loving support of my parents and husband (even if they didn't know the true cause of my mental illness at the time) and with unwavering support from my spiritual team, I navigated mental illness, fear and grief from a very unique perspective. It was the hardest, most traumatic experience of my life... feeling an abyss growing within, a space and void inside myself so large it was unbearable, then dying that one night before having to face and integrate my shadow-self through soul retrieval (an ancient shamanic healing practice that I intuitively knew how to perform). Over time, I discovered that my shadow-self only needed to be shown forgiveness, compassion and love, and although that sounds simple, it was an excruciatingly painful process yet the most rewarding. Just like the idea in art that shadows are needed to really see the play of light, there is always beauty on the other side of pain.

I can't say my life is now void of any stress, anxiety or grief, but I understand, I accept and I have the tools to keep me in balance. I was in the process of writing a memoir, a trilogy called 'Mastering Me', sharing my learning, insights and my experience during my Dark Night of the Soul, when the coronavirus catapulted the world into chaos. I was guided to put this on hold to assist the mass passing of souls through my energy work but to also help the living navigate this crisis too.

I could have created a whole programme based around the content of this book and charged individuals hundreds of pounds to study it, but I wanted this information to be as widely accessible as possible. I therefore settled on writing a book... so here I am! Please don't let your mind or any limiting beliefs deter you from applying the simple steps and process I discovered would bring me back into balance. It doesn't matter if you are not spiritual, if you don't believe, or what culture or religion you follow. It only matters that you want to be happy, healthy and be the best version of you that you can be.

Maybe you have felt lonely self-isolating or under increased pressure home-schooling while trying to keep down a job and have found yourself experiencing parental burnout. Perhaps you have been out fighting for change or in fear and exhausted as a key worker on the front line. Maybe you have lost a business or had a loved one so abruptly taken from you without the chance to say goodbye. Maybe you were struggling with your mental health, an illness, your career or relationships before this pandemic even occurred. You might have thought all was well, but this pandemic has triggered unprocessed ancestral or personal trauma within you. Perhaps you will be reading this book ten years from now when coronavirus is a thing of the past but you are experiencing some other personal crisis or delayed trauma from these times. Whatever your story is, you are welcome here. A life dedicated to 'Mastering Me', I realise now, had a bigger purpose: to help you navigate your own crisis... whatever and whenever that may be. Although long overdue, I am pleased to see a rise in the importance of the mental health agenda, but many people still suffer in silence. I was one of these people, because I felt I couldn't openly discuss the true cause of my personal crisis. So at a time when you may feel helpless, hopeless, lost or alone, let me become a light for you in your darkest hour.

CHAPTER 3

How to Use This Book

This guide book is split into three parts:

* Part 1: Transforming Anxiety and Fear,
* Part 2: Transforming Loss and Grief,
* Part 3: Mastering Your Crown.

Although everyone reading this will be at a different stage in their life, learning and self-development, it is advised that you work through the book in the order laid out in the contents. Although the actual steps contained within this book are simple and straightforward, there is a lot of supporting information surrounding them. You may be tempted to go straight to a particular area of interest, and I do advise against this, because this book is somewhat layered. You may not suffer greatly from anxiety and fear so feel tempted to skip this section, but Part 1 teaches you to how to self-regulate and stabilise yourself from other overwhelming emotions, not just grief. Therefore, Part 1 forms the foundation to progress on to Part 2 of this book.

As you work through this book you will be asked to contemplate certain topics and to complete exercises using pen and paper. Therefore, to help you through this process, I have created a free 'Mastering My Crown; Self Discovery Journal' that you can download from my website: www.emmagholamhossein.com. You can also use it to make key notes or highlight any particular points of interest and to record your thoughts and insights as they arise.

There will be three symbols used throughout this book to help you navigate the information herein with more ease:

 Indicates instructions that will require your physical participation.

 Indicates exercises and instructions that you will need to follow and complete using pen and paper.

 Indicates extra information and ideas to consider, with some top tips.

PART 1: Transforming Anxiety and Fear
The first half of this book from Chapters 4 to 6 is dedicated to transforming anxiety and fear, helping you to navigate the many symptoms and sensations that both bring. Even if your anxiety is mild or you are experiencing very mild stress (and let's face it, who isn't?), this section will help you to bring more balance to your physical body, mind and emotions.

Chapter 4 opens with a discussion about fear, where we look at what happens within the body when we experience it. This key information is fundamental in understanding your anxiety and panic. We also look at the role stress plays in contributing towards ill health and anxiety, the difference between stress and anxiety disorders and the common causes of anxiety, plus some untraditional causes that many people are not aware of.

Chapter 5 describes in detail the steps I used to heal myself from anxiety, panic attacks and PTSD through easy-to-follow instructions. I have named this the '8 Step Sequence', which involves performing eight steps in a set order. The sequence is very quick and simple to do, and at its core is a method of self-regulating your physical body, emotions, mind and energy states. Although the 8 Step Sequence can bring instant relief from acute anxiety and panic symptoms, your body and mind will need time and your commitment to let them heal. To heal basically means to restore to sound 'health', defined by the World Health Organisation (1948) as 'a state of complete physical, mental and social well-being, not merely the absence of disease and infirmity'. To achieve this state, firstly our physical body and its internal environment must be functioning optimally in what we call homeostasis. This internal stability is achieved through the body continually monitoring what is happening inside, checking it has everything it needs to survive, such as oxygen, water, nutrients and the removal of waste, etc. These functions all happen automatically, thankfully—there would be way too much to think about otherwise! I can't remember why I walked into a room some days... Just imagine if you had to remind your stomach to digest your food, tell your heart to beat or your lungs to breathe! In fact, your body is so clever that when something upsets this internal environment, certain changes and adjustments are automatically made to regain its state of dynamic consistency and optimal functioning.

In some instances, these upsets to homeostasis can be quite natural, like when we move from lying to standing, which results in our blood pressure adjusting to suit our position, but in other times these upsets are caused by stress, anxiety and fear. This adaptive response of the body is called 'Allostasis', which describes the maintaining of stability through changes both in physiological regulation and behaviour. When we positively change our behaviour to allow our bodies to remain in homeostasis or a balanced state for longer periods, the body has its own natural healing ability, but so often we don't allow it the time it needs and we quickly look to others to heal our bodies for us. We may then seek help from doctors, physiotherapists and healers etc., often because we have stopped caring and listening to our own bodies' innate wisdom. We eventually lose the ability to hear its cry, so we hand over our power to another. Please don't mistake me, modern medicine is truly amazing and has not only saved but improved countless lives, but I feel there is an overreliance on it. Much ill health could be prevented if we started to care more about ourselves. The 8 Step Sequence is a method by which to do this. No external objects, people or things are needed to perform it, so you will become self-reliant, not dependant on anyone else, which fosters pure autonomy. Just as we have physical health, then, we also have mental health, which is a continuum ranging from good to poor. Like our bodies can become unwell, so can our minds, and there has been masses of research and well-documented evidence that show how the mind and thoughts affect physiology, both positively and negatively. So our internal homeostasis can be affected by our thoughts as well as our external environment. Taking care of our minds, then, becomes equally as important as taking care of our bodies to achieve health. The 8 Step Sequence helps to calm and slow our thoughts too. All you need to do is follow the instructions to perform it.

Chapter 6 is the last of Part 1 and explains why the 8 Step Sequence works. Although physically performing the 8 Step Sequence is extremely simple, the reasons behind why such techniques work are more complex. We look at each step individually and what it does to the body, mind, emotions and subtle energies, exploring both the more scientific anatomy and physiology of the human body and the esoteric energy anatomy. Honouring both helps to bridge the gap between Western medicine and ancient ways of health and healing, because they really are two sides of the same coin.

Once you are experiencing anxiety, panic or fear, it is very difficult to think yourself calm, but once we change our physiology, it is easier to change our thoughts, behaviours and beliefs. The 8 Step Sequence does this even if you aren't aware of the 'whys', but such understanding can be useful, especially if you choose to use any of the steps in isolation. For me, even though my intuitive self knows this sequence is beneficial, as I physically feel and energetically see its positive effects, when I understand the 'whys', it also pleases my conscious logical mind, and then I find I am more willing to perform the sequence even when I feel apathetic and lazy.

Please note that the 8 Step Sequence is NOT a replacement for medication, counselling or any other medical interventions you may be receiving, but it can work alongside such therapies. I do not condone, advise or suggest that you stop taking any prescribed medication without the guidance and agreement of your medical professional team. If you are experiencing any suicidal thoughts, considering harming yourself or another, please seek immediate support. There is a list of helplines and charities that you can contact in Appendix A of this book. Although I didn't take medication for my mental illness, which was my choice, my journey and my path, I'm not suggesting you should follow in my footsteps. Use discernment, use your intuition, and don't be scared to discuss any concerns with your healthcare team about the use of medications, which I know for some is most certainly needed. Just remember that whatever your anxiety and panic trigger is, whatever your fear, you are not alone. I am sure there is someone somewhere in the world who has had a similar experience to you, who feels like you do, so please reach out. For anyone who wishes to link up and connect with me and others who are working through this book, I have set up a free Facebook support group called 'Mastering Your Crown' should you wish to join.

PART 2: Transforming Loss and Grief

The second half of this book, Chapters 7 to 9, is dedicated to transforming loss and grief. Chapter 7 opens with me 'shedding a light' and sharing my story on how I came to understand the differences between them both. We also look at terminology and some common misconceptions.

Chapter 8 explores different types of loss, both physical and symbolic. The outbreak and spread of the coronavirus has not only caused physical death and loss of life, but there has also been loss of what was our 'normal' way of life. Consequently, we have been asked to make changes to our behaviour, limit and sometimes stop social interaction and avoid seeing our family and friends. Many people are losing their jobs, their businesses and their salaries. We have lost our freedom in many ways, and many people don't actually realise that they are in a process of grieving. This will become more apparent when you learn how to assess your own levels of loss by conducting a very simple exercise that involves methodically reviewing all of your major life changes. I have named this 'The Life Review'. Viewing your life in this way can help uncover any unprocessed loss and thus any repressed grief you may be holding. Like myself, you may not even be aware that your current emotional and mental state has been caused by repressed grief until you begin this process.

Chapter 9 is all about grief, and we look at symptoms, types of grief, phases of the grieving process and how complicated grief can arise. Then we explore the method I used to transform my emotions connected to grief, which I simply call 'Letting Go'. Sadly in today's society and certainly within Western cultures, we are not taught or educated on how to process the emotions grief can bring or how best to support a person who is grieving the death of a loved one. It can become an awkward interaction that further alienates the bereaved when they are already feeling fragile and alone. Until we process our own grief, it is very difficult to hold a safe space for another in this emotional state. Whatever loss your grief is caused by, formulating your own 'Life Review' can assist you in more efficiently processing your emotions. This can sometimes be overwhelming, which is why it is important to perform the '8 Step Sequence' alongside the 'Letting Go' process. The sequence will help create stability from within. Then, with calmness and a more balanced physical body and mind, you will better be able to work through your emotional world. You will learn how to become a modern day alchemist, perhaps not turning lead into gold, but transforming your inner world for the better.

I have stated this previously, but I will state it here again: the 'Life Review' and 'Letting Go' process is not a replacement for counselling or any other medical intervention and therapy you may be receiving, but it can work alongside such therapies. I do not condone, advise or suggest that you stop taking any prescribed medication without guidance and agreement from your medical professional team. If you are experiencing grief (acute or chronic), there is a list of resources in Appendix A of this book that may help you.

PART 3: Mastering Your Crown
The final part of this book, Chapters 10 to 11, discusses important additional topics to further aid in your journey of transforming anxiety, fear, loss and grief. Chapter 10 looks at distraction techniques, grounding and earthing, journaling, the benefits of exercise for mental health, nutritional tips, flower essences, Autonomous Sensory Meridian Response (ASMR), adopting a creative outlet for your mental well-being, how to develop good sleep hygiene and how to make lasting behaviour change.

Finally, Chapter 11 looks at the bigger picture, and we explore some basic astrology that enables you to better understand the world we are now living in and why 2020 was the catalyst to profound change here on Earth and for humanity. You will come to know that mastering yourself is not a destination to arrive at but an ongoing process of self-discovery, involving the commitment and dedication to make small, simple, yet repeated behaviour choices that foster well-being. In doing so, you not only learn to become a better version of yourself but you contribute to creating a better world around you.

PART 1:

Transforming Anxiety and Fear

CHAPTER 4

What are Anxiety and Fear?

Understanding Fear

Before we explore anxiety, we must first understand what happens in the physical body when we experience fear, which is the natural and powerful human emotion caused by threat of danger, real or perceived. Fear starts in the mind but triggers a strong physical reaction in the body, an inbuilt reaction crucial to our survival known as the 'fight or flight' response, likely stemming from our evolutionary development. Humans and mammals alike would have needed to hunt for food to survive and might have needed to stand and fight or flee from animals or other environmental dangers. So although fear is generally thought of as a negative emotion, it does serve a purpose because it's what helps keep us safe from real external dangers.

The response to fear all starts in the amygdala (pronounced a-mig-da-la), a region of the brain that is responsible for recognising threat and processing emotions. The amygdala then sends a distress signal to the hypothalamus (another part of the brain), which is commander-in-chief, responsible for controlling many bodily functions including the release of hormones and neurotransmitters that the endocrine system and nervous system respectively distribute around the body to create physical changes. These changes give you a burst of energy and make you become extremely alert; your heartrate and respiration also increase, which enables more blood and oxygen to be pumped around your body faster. Think of these changes like an automatic and super quick warm-up that prepares the body for action! Redistribution of your blood flow occurs from your digestive organs, skin, fingers and toes to your major muscles so you have the strength to run or fight. This is also why you get cold, clammy hands when anxious, due to the blood draining from your extremities, and why you might get an upset stomach due to your digestion slowing. Your pupils also dilate, making your vision sharper, and perhaps objects seem brighter too, enabling you to see any hazards more clearly. I can't help but think of a popular children's tale... 'But Grandmother, what big eyes you have!' said Little Red Riding Hood. 'All the better to see you with, my dear,' replied the wolf.

In recent years, the 'fight or flight' response has come to be known as the 'fight, flight or freeze' response, because in extreme cases of fear, the emotions of shock or terror can arise and render the body motionless. When the conscious thinking part of the brain (the neocortex) perceives a threat too great, too frightening or too distressing, where neither fighting nor escaping is considered a viable option, the self-paralysing 'freeze' response is activated. This inbuilt mechanism can automatically make the brain and body shut down, causing a numbing out where sometimes no pain or fear is felt at all. Some people actually enter an altered reality and dissociate, creating a sense of being detached and disconnected from the world around them. This can happen in extreme cases of fear and trauma but also in times of milder stress. Two physical symptoms that can be particularly unnerving, creating further fear, are depersonalisation and derealisation. Depersonalisation is a sense of being detached from your physical body and your identity so you may find yourself watching yourself like an outsider or having an 'out of body' experience. Derealisation on the other hand is a sense of people, your surroundings and environment feeling unreal or 'not of this world', like a fog or haze blurs the edges between you and the world around you where nothing has any boundaries. Although both can be extremely disturbing to experience, they are just ways the brain tries to protect itself when there is too much going on or when emotions are too intense to process. It's simply another inbuilt safety mechanism of the brain that helps us 'tune out' from overwhelm. When extreme fear and trauma are from an external cause such as an animal predator, it is easier to react via the 'fight or flight' response, but when the conflict and trauma is inside of us where we can't escape our self, there is a tendency to 'freeze' and dissociate, although sex, gender, age and type of trauma also influence which reaction is adopted ($_1$).

The emotional response to fear, however, unlike the physical response, is highly personal. Some people find pleasure in the rush of adrenaline and actively seek excitement, so feeling fear under more controlled conditions can be considered fun, like watching a scary movie or doing a bungee jump. Equally, many people avoid any fear-inducing situations at all costs because the symptoms are too unpleasant and overwhelming for them. Before my mental illness, I guess I was one of those adrenaline junkies. I loved the challenge of skiing down the hardest black run I could find, shouting 'How hard can it be?' to my friends behind me, who were all crazy enough to follow, or the thrill of being thrown about by the crashing waves when kitesurfing. I am much more chilled now though, which is perhaps a result of my mental illness, age, contentment or a combination of them all.

The word fear can also be used to describe something someone is afraid of and is linked to several anxiety disorders or phobias—irrational fears of things that are unlikely to cause any physical harm. It is said that we are born with only two innate fears—the fear of falling and the fear of loud sounds—and that all other fears are evolutionarily influenced to aid in our survival or are learned due to associations or traumatic experiences. However, to understand the simple ways in which the body reacts to fear via 'fight, flight or freeze' is to understand anxiety and panic, because all three are interrelated and one can trigger another. Many people actually come to fear the very natural symptoms of this automatic and inbuilt response, which can in turn cause more anxiety and panic, perpetuating the whole fear cycle.

All about Stress
It is quite normal to feel apprehensive about taking a test or feel nervous about attending a job interview, but when we experience too much or prolonged stress, it can overwhelm us. Just the right amount of stress will help us to perform efficiently at work, thrive socially and live more meaningful lives. To live in this 'optimal-zone' of functioning, we do need some form of stressor, which is a term that describes any cause of stress, either physical or emotional. A stressor is what causes us to take action; it's what causes change to happen. Stressors even include small things such as seeing the pile of ironing build, to an important work deadline. If we didn't have any stressors at all, we would most likely slump into a state of inertia and stasis where nothing would ever get accomplished. So just the right amount of stress is good for us, where we are coping well with any demands, pressure and responsibilities placed upon us. However, when we perceive that demand as too much or we have too many different stressors to cope with all at once, we can be negatively affected. Generally, things we cannot control tend to stress us out the most, like an awkward boss, health concerns and financial issues. Stress can begin to manifest as muscle tension and muscle holding such as a clenched jaw, or feeling unmotivated, unfocused, irritable, impatient, nervous and jumpy. Stress can also impact our physical and mental health by increasing the likelihood of suffering from skin irritations, heartburn, anxiety, high blood pressure, heart disease, obesity and diabetes. Sadly, modern day living with all its worries, excessive responsibilities and tight deadlines no longer means we experience the optimal level of stress but many are overworked, overwhelmed and stressed out.

Neuroscientist Bruce McEwan (2005) created a reasonably new framework for understanding stress, and calls this 'allostatic overload' (2). He describes how when we experience repeated cycles of allostasis—so, overuse of the normal physiological adaptations to regulate the body back to homeostasis—a wear and tear on the body results and eventually leads to the many common diseases of modern-day life. To put it simply, over time our inbuilt fear response, which is intended for emergency use only, gets triggered so much due to everyday stresses that it actually becomes our regular and default response. That is why you may now hear the term 'stress response' used interchangeably with the term 'fear response', because physiologically they cause the same reactions in the body.

If you think of yourself as having a pressure gauge, like the one you find on your water boiler, every time you have a demand to meet or stressor placed upon you (allostatic load), the pressure bar increases, and every time you manage that stressor effectively, the pressure gauge goes down. The bar would constantly oscillate, moving up and down, seeking out an optimal balance point. However, not everyone's pressure gauge is the same. Some work more efficiently and the pressure increase is slow and gradual despite the number of stressors or load experienced, whereas some reach their limits and the emergency red zone very quickly with little or few demands (allostatic overload). The efficiency of your unique pressure gauge all depends on how much stress you experience, your genes, your early development and lifestyle behaviours such as smoking, diet and exercise. Remember that an optimal amount of stress for you could completely overwhelm another; everyone is different, so don't compare yourself to others. Plus, be mindful that at different stages in your life your pressure gauge might change or even become faulty. What you used to cope with easily might now tip you over the edge and put your pressure gauge in the red zone! That's why it is important to get to know yourself better and through self-awareness learn how well you manage any demands, responsibilities and stress placed upon you. Do you revert to unhealthy coping behaviours such drinking, smoking or binge-watching TV? Do you find yourself adopting the same unhelpful emotional response patterns such as frustration, a flared temper or conflict in your relationships? Or is your coping mechanism avoidance, retreating and withdrawing from social engagements and relationships? Do you recognise that your pressure gauge needs a reset and that you might need some TLC and time out to adopt some self-care practices?

Recognising stress and overwhelm is key to managing mental health both long- and short-term, and I use a very simple method to keep myself in check. When I feel the onset of overwhelm from simple daily stressors or my ever-growing 'to-do' list, I feel myself get faster... my thoughts, my movements, my breathing, so I regularly tell myself 'Stop'. I then 'Pause' for a moment, which gives me the space to see if there is a better thought, behaviour or action I can take. Then I tell myself 'Slow', which enables me to 'Respond' from a more mindful and centred place, often making choices that serve me and my body better.

* Stop
* Pause
* Slow
* Respond

Regularly using this simple 'Stop, Pause, Slow, Respond' method will allow you to take charge of your otherwise-automated fear/stress response. As a result the body is less burdened and can return to homeostasis (balance) quicker. You will also find yourself becoming less emotionally reactive. Over time, personal resilience is developed, and you will be able to withstand, adapt and recover from stress more efficiently. Thanks to developments in neuroscience, findings have concluded that the brain is not fixed but can reorganise itself by forming new neural connections. This means that every repetition of thought or emotion reinforces a neural pathway in the brain, so with awareness and conscious effort, we can literally retrain and rewire it. In other words, we can change our ingrained habitual patterns of thinking while experiencing stress, anxiety and fear, instead adopting thoughts and behaviours that diffuse the unpleasant, albeit natural, 'fight or flight' symptoms and sensations instead of fuelling them.

Anxiety and Anxiety Disorders
Getting anxious over a meeting or because you are running late is a normal response to stress, but chronic anxiety does not subside when the stress is removed. There is a constant feeling of unease, worry or tension over something that is about to happen or could happen, which can be accompanied by mild or severe symptoms. Over time, chronic long-term stress and anxiety can develop into anxiety disorders, which are mental illnesses that negatively affect a person's daily life.

Anxiety disorders are a group of related conditions rather than a single disorder, and can include separation anxiety, generalised anxiety disorder (GAD), illness anxiety disorder, panic disorder, agoraphobia, social phobia, obsessive-compulsive disorder (OCD), somatic symptom disorder and post-traumatic stress disorder (PSTD). With most anxiety disorders, even though there is no actual danger or threat to physical safety, the mind can perceive it as such and so the same fear/stress response is activated, over and over again. Over time, this can cause hyperarousal, whereby the body, especially the nervous system becomes overly sensitive to normal, everyday stimulus such as the noise of traffic, a dog barking or bright light. Being easily startled, feeling unnecessarily on edge, being on guard (hypervigilant), having sensitivity to pain, and trouble sleeping are some of the symptoms that may be experienced. Anxiety created by short-term stress can often be managed by using coping strategies, but most anxiety disorders need medication and/or other therapies to manage and control them. Factors that increase your likelihood of experiencing an anxiety disorder include stress, trauma, illness, personality, drug and alcohol use, other mental health disorders and genetics.

Symptoms of Anxiety and Panic
Countless symptoms can be experienced during periods of anxiety, whether from stress or anxiety disorders, with most people only having mild sensations. Feelings of panic, however, are felt more intensely, and we can experience several symptoms all at once in a crescendo and peak. This is otherwise known as a panic attack.

Let's take a look at some of the symptoms of anxiety and panic attacks:

* Sweating
* Trembling
* Dry mouth
* Chest pain, pressure or discomfort
* Shortness of breath
* Dizziness, light-headedness, feeling faint
* Palpitations, fast or irregular heartbeats
* Nausea
* Stomach problems (constipation and/or diarrhoea)
* Tingling, numbness
* Hot flushes, cold chills
* Sense of dread and impending doom
* Negative and/or out of control thoughts
* Thinking there is something very wrong with you
* Sleeping problems
* On constant high alert, watching for signs of danger
* Feeling unreal or detached from your body and surroundings
* Fear of dying
* Feelings of claustrophobia
* Your vision closing in

At a glance, I hope you can begin to see and understand the link between the symptoms of your anxiety/panic and the normal automated changes the body makes from activating the fear/stress response, your symptoms are simply a by-product of this. For some, just understanding this link is enough to reduce any worries over their symptoms, so they begin to have less power. I found naming my sensations out loud sometimes helped ease my mind from further panic. For example, I might say, 'My heart is racing because my brain has interpreted this situation as a threat and thinks I need to run, but there is no threat and I am safe.' Noticing when I felt chest pain, I'd state, 'My shoulders have become tense, which is making my chest muscles contract because I am perceiving danger and bracing for impact, but I'm not in danger, I am safe.' However, although I had all this knowledge of the fear/stress response and understood what was happening to me physically, my conscious thinking brain still found it difficult not to panic about the very real symptoms. My mind would still seem to uncontrollably create further scenarios of danger, perpetuating my anxiety and panic. I came so close to calling an ambulance on several occasions because my symptoms mimicked more severe medical emergencies, but I somehow always managed to rationalise with myself. But for many people, the very real symptoms in the body are just too much for the conscious brain to process, so our mind tells us that there must be something very wrong with us. Herein begins the awful internal mental battle and struggle that so often accompanies anxiety and panic attacks.

The back and forth between logic and emotion, creating even further exhaustion, and then that big crash of tiredness that would follow after regaining some stability and balance. I eventually discovered that positive thinking and affirmations would only get me so far once the fear/stress response had been activated; that's when I was led to target the physical body first through adopting specific behaviours and techniques. I will show you how to do this using the 8 Step Sequence. This will help to reduce your symptoms, so hopefully prevent you from having to withstand that awful internal mental battle. At this point, however, it is important to state that if you do ever experience symptoms of a heart attack or any other serious medical problems, please call the emergency services immediately; do not wait.

Causes of Anxiety and Panic

There are many causes of anxiety and panic, including stress, which we have discussed already. In today's fast-paced living, where we thrive on performance, productivity and perfection, stress may seem inevitable. Even before the threat of coronavirus, our technological age seemed to spin our world faster, putting us under growing pressure to keep up with new social norms and expectations. The endless social media platforms, the instant-gratification culture and desire to have the latest brands, the most advanced gadgets, the most 'likes', and constantly making comparisons to others— the younger generations especially being impacted by such modern ways of living. Many of the older generations have also had to adapt too, with the introduction of technology such as e-mails, passwords and phones for banking, bills and pensions. People from all generations struggle to manage their hectic modern lives and commitments. Although modern-day life has significantly contributed to the rising levels of stress, anxiety and other mental illnesses, the most common causes come from normal life events, many of which can't be avoided since they form part of the natural cycle of life. These include:

* Moving home
* Starting a new job
* Job dissatisfaction
* Unreasonable deadlines
* Excessive workload or pressure
* Illness or injury
* Death of a loved one
* Getting married
* Having a baby
* Divorce
* Loss of a job
* Financial burdens
* Relationship conflicts

Less common causes of stress, anxiety and panic can include traumatic events such as rape, acts of violence, war, terror or theft.

Untraditional Causes of Anxiety and Panic

There are also some untraditional causes of anxiety and panic that many people are still unaware of. Not only are some people less able to cope well under stress (their pressure gauge rises rapidly regardless of the number of stressors) but some 15-20% of the population has been reported to have sensory processing sensitivity (SPS) $(_3)$. This is a term created by psychologists Dr Elaine Aron and husband Dr Arthur Aron in the '90s which describes a personality trait characterised by a high level of sensitivity to external stimuli. Such a highly sensitive person (HSP) who displays SPS would be extremely detail orientated and have a greater capacity to notice more than the average person. They experience their five basic senses of touch, taste, sound, sight and smell at a greater magnitude. They may also be more easily over-stimulated by seemingly mundane things such as a tag on their clothes, hair in their face or white noise, all of which would cause them undue stress and discomfort. They may also display stronger emotions and empathy, another term which is currently trending. Being an empath is not simply being overly sympathetic; it involves being extremely sensitive to the pain and emotions of others. Unlike a HSP, who may just be aware of the emotions of others, empaths will feel the emotions as if they were their own. They absorb both what are seen as positive emotions such as joy and happiness and the more negative, including anxiety, fear, nervousness, agitation, alarm, unease, etc. In the scientific community, a more recent term for such a phenomenon is Emotional Contagion, which suggests that emotions can actually be caught like a flu or virus.

A HSP might not be an empath but most empaths are highly sensitive people, and there are numerous types of empath too, each exhibiting different traits and abilities not within the scope of this book to discuss. To be either a HSP or empath is not a choice; you just simply are, in the same way you can't choose your natural eye colour or where you are born. Some people are aware that they are a HSP or an empath from a very young age or, like me, come to realise this as they mature, grow and come to know and understand themselves on a deeper level. Also, for many who become more consciously aware of themselves, the world around them and the universe in what is often known as a spiritual awakening, they may begin to experience several strange and unexplainable symptoms and sensations. These are sometimes called 'Ascension Symptoms' and are caused by a shifting of your consciousness and subtle energies. Below is a list of symptoms, although by no means exhaustive:

* Unexplained waves of anxiety, edginess and pangs of panic
* A sense of urgency (a feeling of fastness, racing thoughts and movement)
* Sensitivity to toxins and chemicals in foods, beauty products and perfumes
* Sensitivity to noisy, busy environments, extreme temperatures
* Sensitivity to electromagnetic pollution (laptops, mobiles, microwaves, Wi-Fi)
* Spiritual 'flu' symptoms
* Despondency and feeling lost
* Changes in sleeping patterns
* Increased clarity and number of dreams
* Lack of interest in the mundane and disinterest in hobbies you used to enjoy
* Changes in relationships, friendships and social groups
* A desire for radical change
* Sudden changes in beliefs
* Increased synchronicities and meaningful coincidences
* Feeling an overwhelming connection to all people and sentient beings
* Increased intuition empathy and/or emotions
* Increased curiosity, seeking knowledge and understanding
* Sensitivity to Earth changes (quakes, fires, seasonal and 24hr magnetic shifts etc.)
* Sensitivity to planetary movements (lunar cycles, retrogrades, conjunctions etc.)
* Sensitivity to space weather (solar flares, solar winds, comets, etc.)

Please note, many of the Ascension Symptoms listed above can actually mimic symptoms of mild, moderate and severe physical and/or mental health issues, so always seek medical advice to rule out any other possible causes. For example, hyperaesthesia is a medical condition which creates overwhelming sensitivity in one or more of your five basic senses that could be caused by several underlying health issues such as a B-12 deficiency, shingles or nerve damage caused by compression or injury. Hyperthyroidism is a medical condition whereby the thyroid gland produces too much of the hormone thyroxine, accelerating your body's metabolism, causing palpitations, a sense of internal speediness and weight loss. So always err on the side of caution and get yourself checked out. For over a year I suffered from sciatica that became so severe I couldn't sit down. I saw several medical professionals (traditional and alternative) and even had an MRI scan to rule out any serious issues. Thankfully, all was well physically, and I now know that fear and repressed grief were the cause. Once I released these emotions, my sciatica disappeared.

There are also a minority of people who display a sixth sense otherwise known as extrasensory perception (ESP). This minority display abilities such as telepathy (reading another's thoughts), precognition (seeing into the future), retrocognition (seeing into the past), clairvoyance (clear seeing), clairaudience (clear hearing), claircognizance (clear knowing), clairsentience (clear sensing), psychometry (the ability to read information from a person, object or place), etc. All types of ESP contribute to someone's psychic ability. Many times, I have been asked the difference, then, between being psychic and simply being intuitive, and my answer is this: Intuition is an innate ability that all humans have, that hunch or that 'a-ha' moment we have all had when trying to solve a problem. It's instinctively knowing a friend is going to call just before you see their name on your handset or having a gut feeling to drive a certain way home only to find out you missed a hold-up due to an accident. Our gut feelings are not some 'crazy woo-woo' but a part of our Enteric Nervous System (ENS), which we will discuss more later. However, most people's experience of intuition is fleeting and not something they feel they can control. Intuition is subtle and so often missed, but when we learn to listen to it, it can be extremely empowering, like having your own internal GPS system. Being psychic, then, means actively using, further developing and mastering your intuition for a specific purpose. This is when you can begin to tap into your ESP abilities using other parts of the body, not just the gut.

Obviously, as with any skill, some people are more naturally gifted than others, just as a musician, artist or athlete would be, but everyone can certainly learn to harness their intuition and ESP abilities more efficiently with practice. Even fewer people have mediumistic abilities, either from birth or activated later in life, which allow them to channel and communicate with deceased souls, spirits and entities. Such individuals might not be HSPs, empaths or intuitive at all. There is no one-size-fits-all; each person is unique, with their own gifts, abilities, strengths and weaknesses. Although such labels are needed for conceptual understanding, it is far too simplistic a view to box people into this category or that. Thankfully though, the terms are becoming more widely accepted and less taboo thanks to the developments in parapsychology and neuroscience. However, it is no coincidence that as humanity enters a period of great spiritual awakening and rise in consciousness (we discuss why in Part 3), the world has been and continues to be in the midst of a mental health epidemic. I believe the two are intrinsically linked. Latent abilities that have been forgotten and laid dormant within us are being remembered and activated. When one awakens in consciousness and parts of the psyche, brain, subconscious memory and DNA become activated, this can in turn create many strange symptoms and changes within the body as these new abilities integrate. So although anxiety and fear, loss and grief may seem like two distinct and separate issues—and they can be—I came to discover that my anxiety and panic attacks were caused by my innate sensitivity, spiritual awakening and fear of my growing psychic abilities. My PTSD was caused by my traumatic spiritual experience (my Dark Night of the Soul) and repressed grief, both of which triggered within a fear of death and dying commonly known as 'death anxiety' but more accurately termed thanatophobia. Due to our very human nature, most—but not all—people fear death in some way, whether that be the cessation of your own existence or the death of a loved one. There is much debate as to whether fear of death is an instinctual or learned response, but either way, transforming your anxiety and grief can help you find some peace of mind in accepting your mortality. If, however, you are one of the minority who do not fear death and your anxiety is caused by other triggers, this book can also help you to manage your symptoms better, creating more balance within.

CHAPTER 5

The 8 Step Sequence

What is the 8 Step Sequence?
The 8 Step Sequence is a series of eight techniques that help bring balance to the body, mind, emotions and subtle energies. At its core, it is a method of self-regulation that is simple and quick to perform. Therefore, the 8 Step Sequence can be used in many scenarios, such as at the onset of a panic attack to reduce symptoms, if you are feeling anxious about an upcoming event such as a job interview or hospital appointment, or if you have been shielding and feel apprehensive or nervous about going out into society again. The sequence will help keep your nerves at bay so you can stay aware but not overstimulated. Think of it as a tool that, with practice, you will come to master and, like a faithful friend, can turn to in times of need.

You may find that you use the 8 Step Sequence more frequently initially, during periods of real anxiety and overwhelm, then as you become more balanced in mind, body, emotions and subtle energies, you may feel called to use it less. However, try not to stop indefinitely, because your symptoms may creep back and you will think the sequence hasn't worked. That is what I have seen most in my clients: they start feeling better, so stop. Ideally, the sequence should be used as an ongoing method of self-care to help you maintain a sense of physical stability, emotional balance and confidence. Like regular check-ups at the dentist help to prevent more complex problems from occurring, practising the 8 Step Sequence regularly, even when you feel well, will help keep you more stable as you journey through life's ups and downs.

Although I discovered the techniques more organically throughout my mental illness, I have formulated them into a sequence that, when followed in this order, has greater benefits. The techniques that make up the 8 Step Sequence are as follows:

THE 8 STEP SEQUENCE

1) Psoas Shake

2) Thymus/Adrenal Gland Reset

3) Vagus Nerve Stimulation

4) Sensing

5) Hara Breathing

6) Medulla Hold

7) Crystalline Matrix Alignment

8) Figure 8 Pose

How to Perform the 8 Step Sequence

The most effective way to bring calm and balance to your body, mind, emotions and subtle energies is to complete this sequence of techniques in order, daily or as frequently as possible. Please don't wait until you feel anxious or overwhelmed to perform the sequence; begin by practising when you are calm so you can familiarise yourself with it, also building a habit. It takes no more than ten minutes to complete, but if you wish to spend extended amounts of time on any one technique, you can. You can also perform each step as a standalone exercise, if you wish. However, the most effective results come from performing the 8 Step Sequence in its entirety and in the order listed, at least once a day. You don't need any specific equipment; your willingness to be open-minded and follow the instructions are all that you need. I do suggest, however, being sat upright in a chair with your feet flat on the floor, ideally somewhere quiet, although that is not absolutely necessary. Quietness does aid in allowing your awareness to rest on the process taking place and allow any feedback between the body, mind and subtle energies to be observed more easily. As you get more confident and efficient at performing the sequence, you could practise it in different environments, becoming more prepared for when you may come to need it. The power of the 8 Step Sequence lies in its simplicity, as no external objects, people or things are needed to perform it. There is no dependency on anything or anyone else, which fosters pure autonomy.

However, I appreciate that learner needs can differ; therefore, you can find a video demonstration of me performing the 8 Step Sequence in the free 'Mastering Your Crown' Facebook group and, for a small extra fee, an audio download of the instructions on my website: www.emmagholamhossein.com. Both are additional learning aids and should not replace working through the entirety of this book.

As previously mentioned, the 8 Step Sequence should take no longer than ten minutes to perform. However, I understand that lack of time is the number one biggest barrier to adopting health-promoting behaviours. Therefore, plan to perform the 8 Step Sequence and make it part of your daily routine, possibly after brushing your teeth or—as silly as this sounds—while on the toilet. I often hear people say 'I haven't got time' or 'I don't have time', but what they are actually saying is... 'I am not willing to replace anything that I currently fill my time with or adjust my current lifestyle in any way.' Because when something becomes a priority to someone, time can always be found, and as a wise person once said, 'If you don't find time for health, you will soon have to find time for illness.' Regardless of how busy your life is, you always have a choice. The question is 'Do you respect, like and consider yourself worthy enough to give yourself just ten minutes of your time a day to help improve your health?' If the answer is no, I suggest asking yourself why. If you are in better physical health and in a more stable emotional and mental state, life becomes easier and you can more positively connect to those around you... Your children, family, partner and co-workers, etc. Therefore, if you can't yet do it for yourself, do it for them. The people you love deserve to see the best version of you. Try setting your alarm ten minutes earlier every day, or each time you feel pulled to check your social media, pause and remember that you won't get that time back... Maybe perform the 8 Step Sequence instead.

 In summary, guidelines for performing the 8 Step Sequence are as follows:

Equipment:	A chair
Frequency:	Daily (or as many times as needed)
Duration:	10 minutes
Instructions:	Follow in set order

You may also like to monitor yourself before and after performing the 8 Step Sequence, rating whether your anxiety or overwhelm reduces. Use a simple scale such as 1 (lowest anxiety) to 10 (highest anxiety).

The 8 Step Sequence Instructions

STEP 1: Psoas Shake

 Adopt an easy standing position and hold on to the back of a chair, the wall or a stable structure for balance. Then lift one leg only about two inches from the floor, slightly flex the foot (lift your toes towards your head) and proceed to shake your leg. The knee should not repetitively lock, and the movement should initiate from up at the hip, where you let the leg lengthen away from the body. Start gently, and as the leg starts to release, use a slightly faster shake that feels rhythmical and vibrates up the torso like a tremor. Imagine you are trying to shake something off your heel. However, please ensure that you are not just shaking your ankle. In fact, if your ankle is too lax and floppy, it will hinder your ability to fully unlock your psoas muscle. You are not kicking the leg either, which would lock out the knee joint and could cause damage to the ligaments and tendons. You are creating a vibration that travels up the leg muscles to reach the bottom muscle. Once you have completed the exercise with both legs, if you wish, you can also shake your arms in the same manner, and whole body too.

 You might also like to add a very gentle bounce and stomp through the feet. Please keep the knees soft and supple to avoid any impact and unnecessary force through the joints. You might also like to accentuate this movement even more by really shaking the whole body, moving freely, flowing, swaying, shaking, rocking, uninhibited by your conscious mind. I must say I initially found this very difficult, firstly because my body had become so rigid, stuck in fear and trauma, and secondly because I was conscious of what this may have looked like. Losing inhibition was a huge barrier for me to overcome. Interestingly, when I was well and healthy in the mind, I wouldn't have thought twice about letting it rip on the dance floor on a night out, but due to becoming frozen in trauma, I even found shaking a limb a challenge. So my advice would be, just start small, just allow yourself to shake the legs, then the rest will come.

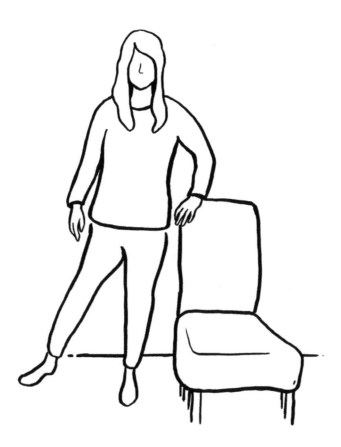

Step 1. Psoas Shake

STEP 2: Thymus and Adrenal Gland Reset

 Place your right palm at the centre of your chest, fingers pointing diagonally up towards your left shoulder. Then gently slide your palm slightly to the left side until you feel the edge and heel of the hand (known as the Mount of Venus) sink into the depression at the centre of your chest and sternum. Using downward sweeps repeatedly soothe the area between your collar bone and middle of your chest (the location of your thymus gland) with your Mount of Venus five to eight times. (2a.) Now slide both palms towards your waist then behind to your mid-back, fingers pointing down and towards the line of the belly button (umbilicus). Keep your palms gently rested in position (the location of your adrenal glands), then in downward sweeps, using the Mount of Venus and edge of the heel of your hand, gently soothe your adrenal glands. Again, five to eight times will suffice. (2b.) Now unite the palms together at the front of the chest and extend the arms straight in front of you, gently allowing your shoulders to round forwards. As you begin to inhale, start to open your arms wide so the chest expands and protrudes. (2c.) As you exhale, keeping the arms straight, reverse the movement, bringing your palms back to unite.

 As you inhale, this movement takes your upper spine (thoracic vertebrae) into extension, and as you exhale, curling forward, you are moving into gentle thoracic flexion. If you've ever done yoga or Pilates, you will be familiar with these terms. Although the movements described above directly assist in soothing the thymus gland and deactivating the adrenal glands, I found it powerful to state 'relax' or 'stand-down' as I performed them. The movement (extension and flexion of the thoracic spine) described above should not be forced or pushed past your normal range of motion, and it can also be performed sitting or standing. It is also worth noting that for anyone who is experiencing depression without anxiety and/or panic symptoms, I suggest performing the Thymus Tap instead. You still locate the thymus gland by gently sliding your palm slightly to the left side of your chest until you feel the Mount of Venus sink into the depression at the centre of your sternum. But instead of using downward sweeps, gently tap the area with all fingertips and thumb closed together like a beak.

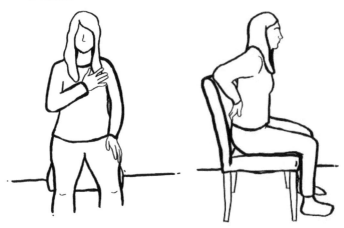

Step 2. Thymus Reset   **Step 2a. Adrenal Gland Reset**

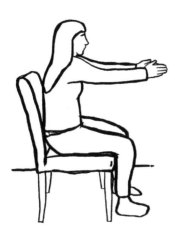   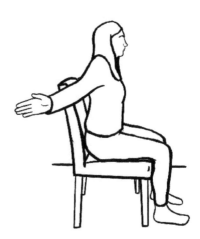

**Step 2b. Adrenal Gland
Massage**   **Step 2c. Thymus Massage**

STEP 3: Vagus Nerve Stimulation

 Gently use your index finger and thumb to massage your earlobes for several seconds and then begin to gently draw them downwards. Use gentle pinching and pulling movements. (3a.) With the tips of your three middle fingers, begin to draw small circular movements just behind the earlobes, where you will feel a small depression. Continue with these slow, circular, rhythmical movements towards the edge of your jaw, then continue straight down the neck to just above the collarbone. To finish, use downward sweeps stimulating the skin of the neck, by holding your three middle fingers rigid and drawing the skin down as you slowly lengthen and lift your chin. Be sure to thoroughly work the right side of your ear and neck.

 You may also like to introduce humming, singing or even chanting a sound such as 'Om' when you do this. You can do this technique anywhere, on the bus, in the office, during a meeting but you might want to keep humming, singing or chanting to when you are alone or you may have some funny looks. Please don't be alarmed if you feel a burning sensation at the skin and site you have stimulated (ears and neck). This is superficial fascia (an important connective tissue of the body) being released.

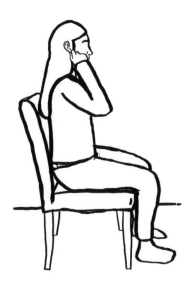

**Step 3. Vagus Nerve
Stimulation – Ears**

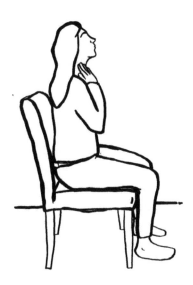

**Step 3a. Vagus Nerve
Stimulation – Neck**

STEP 4: Sensing

 Close your eyes and bring your attention to your body, firstly by finding the chair underneath you, becoming aware of the weight of your body being supported by it. Feel and become aware of the area between your thighs, at the very top where they meet your bottom. Allow yourself to explore that more, perhaps check the weight of your body in the chair—is it equal in both bottom cheeks and hips?

Maybe you can sense that your lower back is being supported by the chair too, or maybe your spine is erect all by itself. Now take all of your attention and focus to your knees. Pay attention to your kneecaps and the backs of them too. Feel into the creases, the line of fold behind both knees. What can you sense? Is there creaking, stiffness, rigidity, or is there suppleness and fluidity? Now feel into your feet. Find them with your awareness, and sense whether they feel cool, warm, icy or burning, relaxed or tense. Explore your feet as much as possible. Can you feel any pressure from shoes or socks, if you have them on? Can you feel the carpet or floor tiles pressing against your soles? What texture can you feel? Is it smooth, rough or spiky? Explore your toes, your heels, the balls of your feet too. Sense them in relation to the rest of your body.

 As you develop this sensing ability, you might like to try it with your eyes open. With practice, it can be done anywhere. Most people can sit in a chair with their feet flat on the floor, but if you are bedridden or physically unable to do this, please visualise your feet making contact with the ground. You might even like to ask another to physically touch your feet, which will help you connect to them and also ground your energy. If you enjoy this practice and want to spend more time sensing, explore other body parts too, but your bottom, knees and feet should always be the main areas of focus. If you are experiencing severe trauma and/or PTSD, I suggest connecting to your bottom, knees and feet, but instead of sensing the rest of your body, tap it down instead. Use the palms of your hands to pat down your arms, torso and legs to give you a sense of physicality, feel that your body has a boundary and an endpoint.

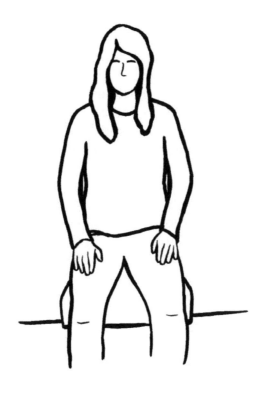

Step 4. Sensing

STEP 5: Hara Breathing

 Now you are present, focused and aware, place your hands one on top of the other just below your belly button. Allow your shoulders to relax, melting away from your ears, then allow your jaw to loosen. Bring your tongue to gently rest at the roof of the mouth, where you will feel it gently pressing behind your front teeth, allowing your lips to softly part. Then take your attention to the tip of your nose. Allow yourself to feel the air as it enters through your nostrils. Explore that sensation further, sensing whether the air is cool or warm, whether you have equal airflow; you might even feel one nostril is slightly blocked. Now follow the flow of air with your conscious awareness through the nostrils and to the back of the throat on each in-breath, allowing yourself to become more relaxed with each out-breath. Continue to follow the flow of air through the nostrils and to the back of the throat. As you continue relaxing into this breathing, allow the breaths to become slightly longer, especially the out-breath. Now continue to consciously follow the flow of air from the nose to the throat but allow it to continue into the chest. You can imagine your chest like a contained box, with a top, a bottom and four sides. With each in-breath, allow this box to get bigger, expanding on all four sides.

As you see the box getting bigger, your chest expanding more deeply, you naturally begin to draw in more air. But don't let your awareness skip straight to your chest each time. Remember to follow the flow of air, always starting each in-breath at the tip of the nose, taking it to the back of your throat, then into the chest. Continue with this breathing until you witness your breath and your chest rhythmically lifting and falling on its own. Like naturally flowing waves that softly break against the shoreline and then gently pull back, over and over. Be mindful that, as you take in more air and oxygen, it can make you feel a little light-headed, so don't force yourself. Always aim for your out-breath to be longer than your in-breath, and there is no need to hold in-between breaths. Now, as you witness your chest start to expand with your in-breath, see the base of the box gently open like a valve, and as it does, allow your awareness to travel deeper into your abdomen. Explore this space, feel for any tightness or restriction; you may even witness emotions begin to arise. All the time, just allow the breathing to continue, keeping your focus, your internal gaze and awareness at your lower tummy. Relaxed and rhythmically, you are now taking your awareness with each in-breath all the way to your lower tummy.

Now, on your next out-breath, gently draw your tummy muscle in towards your spine, then on your next inhalation, feel the tummy naturally expand. Allow this breathing to simply continue. Always take your awareness to the tip of your nose at the start of each in-breath, follow that breath to the back of the throat, into the chest, feeling it expanding as your awareness drops into your lower tummy. Then, as the out-breath begins, draw the lower tummy muscle in, watch the chest deflate. Continue to rhythmically breathe in this manner, just allowing your awareness to rest at your lower tummy.

 Eventually, when you have mastered this, you will begin to sense the in-breath initiating from the lower tummy. Almost like your belly is breathing for you. Once you feel this shift, explore that sensation, explore that feeling coming from deep inside your lower tummy. See this area deep within you, like a small sphere of pulsating energy breathing for you. If this shift doesn't happen automatically, consciously take the in-breath to meet with your hands, which are placed one on top of the other at your lower tummy. This is the hardest step of the 8 Step Sequence and it will take practice and time to master.

Since I have been performing this type of breathing for a very long time, it tends to take me two or three breaths to connect fully with my lower abdomen. However, when I was anxious or busy in the mind, I couldn't always connect to it, and when I did, it took me maybe 40 to 60 breaths. I never really counted. It wasn't important how many breaths it took or the duration of the in- and out-breaths; it was always about how I felt once I got there. You will feel such a deep sense of peace, you cease trying and simply become one with the breath or the breath becomes you... it's hard to distinguish at that point. However, please, please, please, don't worry if you can't reach such a state or if you feel you are doing it wrong. It takes practice. But more importantly, don't think that it's not worth doing if you struggle with it initially, because there are so many benefits to this technique. You wouldn't expect to run a marathon without training for it first. Be gentle with yourself, be kind to yourself. Be willing to get it wrong, but just don't give up. Also, don't be alarmed if you begin to feel warmer as you do this or if emotions arise. Allow them to come, allow them to go, and just continue to bring your awareness back to following the flow of your breath.

As with all types of breathing techniques, some people experience dizziness. This means you are taking in too much oxygen and not letting out enough carbon dioxide. It really is important not to force the breath, not to gulp the air you are breathing in, and to allow your exhalation to become progressively longer than your inhalation. It may seem a lot to think about, but it's like driving a car... although that's probably not a good example! I can hear my mum saying, 'I don't drive, so that's not helpful to me!' So just like any new skill you learn, no matter your age, repetition and commitment to practice is key.

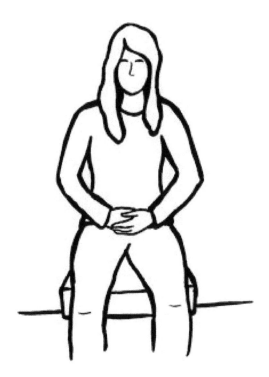

Step 5. Hara Breathing

STEP 6: Medulla Hold

 Place both palms on the back of the head at the base and protruding part of the skull; this is called the occipital bone. Simply hold your hands in position without any movement, index fingertips touching and little fingers pointing upward. Continue taking several long, slow, deep breaths as you hold.

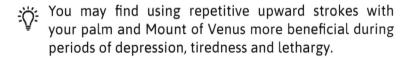 You may find using repetitive upward strokes with your palm and Mount of Venus more beneficial during periods of depression, tiredness and lethargy.

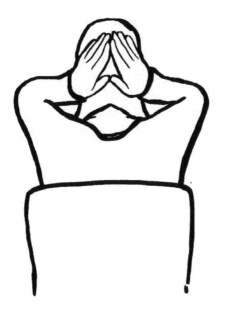

Step 6. Medulla Hold

STEP 7: Crystalline Matrix Alignment

 Cross your arms, placing both hands on the front of opposite shoulders at the end of your collarbone (the acromioclavicular joint) and hold for several seconds. (7a.) Uncross your arms then place both hands on the side of each hip. Again, hold for several seconds. (7b.) Cross arms, placing both hands on opposite knees, hold for several seconds. (7c.) Then finally, uncross arms, placing both hands across the bridge of the feet at the ankles, hold for several seconds.

 Some people will favour right arm over left, while others will favour left over right. Just allow yourself to feel comfortable and do what intuitively and instinctively comes, without thinking too much about it. The body's energetic circuitry is changing constantly, so one day you might find yourself right over left, another day you might feel more comfortable to use left over right. Don't be limited by the mind or learned behaviour, be willing for your body and intuition to lead you.

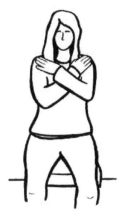

**Step 7. Crystalline Matrix
Alignment – Shoulders**

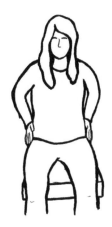

**Step 7a. Crystalline Matrix
Alignment – Hips**

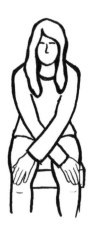

**Step 7b. Crystalline Matrix
Alignment – Knees**

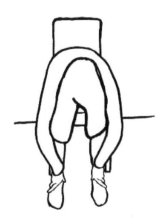

**Step 7c. Crystalline Matrix
Alignment – Ankles**

STEP 8: Figure 8 Pose

Cross one foot over the other at the ankle. Don't think too much about this, just perform that movement now. If you find you have placed the right foot over the left ankle, now cross your left wrist over your right, allowing them to rest in your lap with palms facing down. If you crossed your left ankle over your right, you should cross your right wrist over left. In either case, your wrists and ankles should be opposites. Now direct your toes together and allow your heels to slightly rise off the floor. The balls of the feet remain in contact with the floor. Allow your shoulders to melt down, and hold this position for several breaths.

As with the Crystalline Matrix Alignment, some people will favour right over left ankles and wrists, while others will favour left over right. Just allow yourself to feel comfortable and do what intuitively and instinctively comes without thinking too much about it. The main thing to remember is the ankles and wrists should be crossed in opposite directions. Working this way allows for energy changes and means that the movement may differ slightly each time you perform the Figure 8 Pose. (8a.) If you are an earth empath who needs a respite from Earth changes, perform the Mastering Me Loop instead by placing the soles of your feet together then allowing your knees to open in a diamond shape. Next, place your palms together and remain in this position for several breaths or for as long as you feel you need.

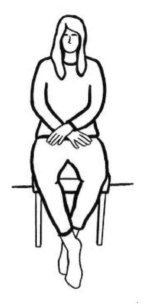

Step 8. Figure 8 Pose

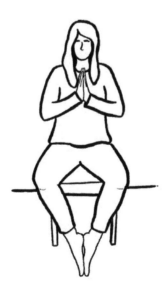

Step 8a. Mastering Me Loop

CHAPTER 6

Why the 8 Step Sequence Works

So now you have discovered just how simple the 8 Step Sequence is to perform, we are going to explore why it works. This will be highly interesting for some, especially if you have an inquisitive mind like mine and like to understand how things function, specifically the human body, the mind and what I call 'energy anatomy'. Although I have simplified the following information, some may find it a little... hmmm... how can I say... scientific! However, please know that you do not need to remember any of what you are about to read in order for the sequence to work. You don't even have to understand it, but I have included it within this book because I want to cater for all levels of ability and interest. So don't let reading the complex 'whys' put you off from performing the extremely simple 8 Step Sequence.

STEP 1 – Psoas Shake to Keep Connected

The psoas (pronounced 'so-as' so drop the 'p') is a very special muscle deep within our core, which—like all muscles—can be greatly affected by anxiety and fear. However, what makes this muscle more significant than others is its location and function... it's the only muscle in the entire body that connects our upper body to our lower body, our spines to our legs. Although it is traditionally thought of as one of the muscles in the hip flexor group (bring your knee up to your chest and you've activated it), it's so much more. It has an important role as a postural muscle because it aids in spinal and pelvis stabilisation, while also being a powerful mind-body-energy connector. Technically there are two psoas muscles, the psoas major and the psoas minor, both of which start at the last thoracic vertebrae (T12) and the first lumbar vertebrae (L1)—but finish up at different places. The psoas major attaches to all the lower vertebrae and crosses the hip joint to end inside the top of the thigh bone, whereas the psoas minor attaches to the front of the pelvic bone, so does not cross the hip. When people talk of the psoas muscle, it is generally the psoas major that is being referred to, in fact over half of the population don't even have a psoas minor muscle. As you can see from Diagram 1, you have a psoas muscle on each side of the pelvis.

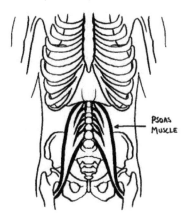

Diagram 1. The Psoas Muscle

But before we get into the nitty-gritty as to why you should get in touch with your psoas muscle and 'shake it, baby, shake it', I'll give you a little backstory! I was maybe six weeks into my PTSD and I was still fighting with my severe panic attacks and dissociation (a feeling of being disconnected from my body), but I suddenly felt inclined to try and meditate. I didn't even manage five minutes before *whoosh*, my internal alarm system sounded off and my body jolted into a panic. It was strange, because it was the first time I had been in my meditation room since my Dark Night of the Soul and thus the onset of my PTSD, but although my body was firing off, part of my awareness managed to hear my intuition. I felt that awful drop in my gut then knot in the pit of my stomach;

my heart was racing, my insides and limbs trembling, but my head hadn't followed my body. It managed to remain calm and indifferent in my meditation space, and it was like having a foot in two different realities. My body so wanted to spring to its feet, the instinct to flee the room was so great, but something made me stay. I then saw, for the first time in what felt like forever, Lone-Wolf, my spirit guide, appear in his full ceremonial attire, war bonnet of feathers swaying around as he danced and stomped his feet. He had always been a man of very few words, rather stoic and serious-looking, but his body language suggested I join in. I said, 'You want me to dance?!', all confused and annoyed at his seeming lack of concern. I mean, couldn't he see I was in turmoil on the verge of a major panic attack? Why on earth would I want to dance? Plus, where had he been these last few months at my darkest hour?

Part of my being was being pulled to react as I normally would have, while another part of me instantly knew I was being shown another way.

It's a very funny story actually—not for this book, sadly—but I came to learn how Lone-Wolf and the men of our Native Tribe would perform a Ritual War Dance before going into battle. The stomping and repetitive foot movements thrust into the ground would help to transform the emotion of fear into strength and power. They would mimic certain animals too, moving and freeing their bodies to help them connect to the Great Spirit of Mother Earth, grounding their energy into a fully present and embodied state. I wasn't at all in the mood for dancing, although if I had done so, I would have probably felt significantly better, but I just couldn't, I was too frozen. Dancing for me had usually been out of joy and happiness, both emotions I was no longer feeling, or because music had stirred something within me and inspired me to move my body. But since I couldn't even listen to music due to it overstimulating my sensitised nervous system, I was shown how I could simply shake out the fear instead, no music needed. So that's what I did. It almost sounds too simple doesn't it? However, once I began, I instantly started to feel the positive effects of transforming my own fear into power. When I started to really feel the emotions moving within me, I learned to direct the fear out of different parts of my body. I had no set pattern, I literally just shook, wobbled, jiggled, shuddered and vibrated my hands, arms, legs and bum as if I wanted to flick something off me, out of me even. As I did this I felt empowered. I was taking back control and now had a method to move myself through the 'freeze' response I had been stuck in, albeit unconsciously. This was the start of me developing the 8 Step Sequence, even if I didn't know it at the time.

So now let's briefly explore why this method of shaking out fear works and why targeting the psoas is also needed. You may yourself have seen a dog perform this very natural response to calm a stimulated nervous system. Every time I come home from walking my dog, regardless of whether he is wet or not, after I remove his harness, he immediately shakes his whole body. This is to reset his nervous system, release tension, stress and/or any remaining excitement. In humans, tremors can be associated with many nervous system disorders but can also be quite natural, like after holding a deep squat for any length of time, when your teeth chatter in the cold or if you've had too much coffee. Stress, anxiety and fear can also cause your body to make involuntary tremors... you know, when your hands tremble before walking into that big interview or when your knees judder and weaken after you've been startled.

However, especially where fear and trauma are concerned, we have been taught and conditioned to repress this tremor. Showing signs of fear can be seen as a weakness, so we try to hold it together to seem physically robust and unmoving. This has hindered a very natural way to dissipate the effects of the 'fight, flight or freeze' response. Panic and fear then get trapped in the body, getting pushed down into our muscles, joints, cells and subconscious, which can eventually manifest as physical and mental issues. So shaking out fear allows the uncomfortable sensations and emotions that it brings to flow unhindered through us. We can actually process our stress hormones (adrenaline, noradrenaline, cortisol, etc.) positively through movement.

While this method of shaking was extremely powerful for me, one day I became aware that the fear sensations wouldn't travel through my hip. My intuition told me 'my psoas muscle is hypertonic', a term which means too much or excessive (hyper) tone (tonic) or tension. Funnily enough, although it was my own intuition that told me this, I had to Google its meaning because my brain was mush—it was like my memory had been deleted... another wonderful symptom of PTSD. This is when I came to realise the connection between the psoas muscle, fear and trauma, the root chakra and my inability to feel safe. As you now know, the psoas muscle is deep within the pelvis, the bridge between our upper body and lower body. Well, when that muscle is in a constant state of contraction (hypertonic) and not in a relaxed tone (pliable and supple), like a drawbridge that has become stuck in the air, energy and emotions cannot easily pass from the torso, into the legs and out through the knees and feet. It also becomes more difficult to feel the strong grounding and nurturing presence of the Earth's energy underneath us. Then, over time, a disconnection between our body and mind grows. We shift from being fully present and embodied to living in our mind space constantly. Just like a fuse can blow, over time we fail to earth our own energy, so it builds and can cause our electromagnetic powerhouses—our brain (minds) and heart (emotions)—to short circuit. Welcome, mental illness and physical malfunctions! The psoas muscle has also become misused in modern day life due to prolonged hours spent sitting, which can lead to a shortened and tight muscle. Over time this can create lumbar lordosis, a forwardly tilted pelvis creating excessive curvature of the lumbar spine, bringing with it poor posture, back pain and pelvic instability. So for many, the muscle is already in a vulnerable state, even before any additional anxiety and fear are experienced.

In summary then, a hypertonic psoas muscle can be caused by repetitive stress, fear, trauma, through poor posture and injury. Each person is unique in how and where their body holds that tension and trauma, so each person will have different dysfunctional movement patterns too. Most people think that stretching an overly tight psoas muscle will solve all the problems, but you can't effectively stretch a permanently contracted muscle. You need to release it first and unlock the cause of its dysfunction. If you have any mobility or spinal issues, or have chronic pain, I do suggest seeking out a body worker who can conduct a comprehensive assessment on you to correct any muscular imbalances.

In Western esoteric traditions, we have a subtle energy layer just off our physical body called the Etheric Body. Think of the 'Ready Brek' man! However, unlike the somewhat-fixed physical body, the subtle energy body is transient and fluid. Connected to our etheric body we also have centres of energy commonly known as chakras that emanate and absorb energy in a somewhat spiral and toroidal fashion. You may have heard of the seven very well-known chakras, namely the crown, third eye, heart, solar plexus, sacral and root, but we have so many more. They don't always sit neatly in place either; I've seen many people whose chakras are not located where we are led to believe they should be. It is proposed that each chakra correlates to a bundle of nerves, particular glands of the body, certain emotions and an area of our physical life. While I can understand how such theories have been formulated, the chakra systems are actually much more complex, but for the purpose of this book, I am going to adopt the simplified and most well-known explanations. The root chakra, which should be located at the perineum (that area of skin between your anus and vagina in women and testes in men), is connected to our adrenal glands (the fight or flight glands), so also oversees our sense of safety and security. For example, having a job that provides financial support so we have a home to protect us and food to nourish us... the basics of survival, then. A poorly functioning, stuck, underactive or closed root chakra could manifest as a lack of safety, belonging and connection, not only to our own body, but in relationships with others too.

So we may begin to feel lost, lose our sense of purpose and disengage from society.

In extreme fear, the root chakra can become completely inverted, like mine did, and I can only postulate that this is what happens when stuck in the 'freeze response'. A healthy root chakra, at macro level, is feeling safe as a species on our planet, where Mother Earth is our home and can provide for us.

As an individual, at micro level, it's feeling nurtured, loved and safe within our physical body: the home for our consciousness, mind and emotions. So, the root chakra and the psoas muscle have very similar functions, fostering connection to our home— albeit one energetic and one physical in nature. One affects the other; they are interconnected. The foundation to the root chakra actually forms from birth until the age of about two years old, so a complex mix of biological, genetic, emotional and physical factors play a part in its functioning.

So now you know your 'whys', all you need to do is 'shake it, baby, shake it' your whole body, but focus on your legs and hips so the shake and vibration travels up into the groin and to the psoas muscle.

Step 2 – Thymus and Adrenal Gland Reset to Pull Rank
Both the thymus gland and adrenal glands form part of the endocrine system: the chemical messenger system of the body, which oversees our hormones. They basically tell our body what to do, when to do it and for how long. Other endocrine glands include the thyroid, parathyroid, pituitary, pineal and hypothalamus, while the pancreas, ovaries and testes form part of this system too but are organs not glands. The most fascinating thing about this system is its negative feedback control, which means it regulates itself, much like how the thermostat in your home works. If the temperature drops below a certain level then the thermostat kicks in to increase the temperature. Once an optimal temperature is reached, it

turns off again. So when some change in your body is detected, a hormone is released to regulate that change—clever, eh?

Thymus Gland Reset

As you know I like geeky facts, so here's one to start: the thymus gland gets its name from the thyme leaf because it vaguely resembles its shape... pyramidal with two lobes. As you can see from Diagram 2, it is found underneath your breast bone (sternum) towards the middle of your chest, next to the outer sac that covers your heart (pericardium). Although the thymus is considered part of the endocrine system as the gland releases hormones, it is also a lymphoid organ so forms part of the lymphatic immune system, along with the spleen, bone marrow, lymph nodes, fluid, skin and appendix, all of which are responsible for fighting off pathogens such as viruses, bacteria and other microbes that can enter the body and multiply, causing infection. When our immune system or body's defence mechanism is weak or not working properly, germs and other abnormal cells in the body can accumulate and cause disease. Smoking, alcohol and poor nutrition—the most common unhealthy coping strategies for stress, might I add—can all weaken the immune system, but so can stress. A constantly activated fear/stress response, so being in 'flight or fight' mode, greatly reduces the body's ability to fight off foreign bodies since the immune response is suppressed in favour of dealing with the perceived danger.

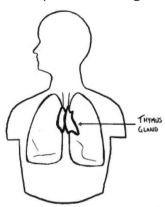

Diagram 2. Location of the Thymus Gland

The thymus gland's main job is to store and mature T-lymphocytes (T-cells) which are our 'killer' white blood cells, those critical to the adaptive immune system, which actually lock on to, attack and destroy infected cells. All lymphocytes begin their life in bone marrow, some stay there to become B-cells, whose job it is to produce antibodies, while others migrate to the thymus to become our super-duper 'killer' T-cells. 'B' for bone, 'T' for thymus... so simple even I can't forget that one! Interestingly, the thymus gland is largest in children when the immune system is developing and the T-cells spend time maturing there. Just like how only the best students graduate, only competent T-cells get to leave the thymus gland after stringent testing, while most are destroyed. Then as we age, the thymus kicks back, puts its feet up and starts slowing down, declining in function and in size (called involution). It actually shrinks, becoming more fatty tissue, and by about 65 years of age, it is said that the thymus stops making T-cells all together.

The link between thymus involution and aging is well documented and research has suggested that the decline in thymus function correlates to a decline in the immune system, along with the subsequent ineffective defence against disease such as inflammation and cancers that occur more prominently as we age. Interestingly, in 2019 researchers from the Monash Biomedicine Discovery Institute identified the factors responsible for this age-related decline of the thymus, which has opened up a whole new area of study that aims to find ways to reverse this decline and effectively turn the thymus back on again so that greater T-cell production resumes (4). However, until hard science can tell us more, it's important to keep the thymus functioning to the best of its ability for as long as biologically possible ourselves.

There is actually a well-known ancient energy technique that originates from India and Ayurvedic medicine (one of the world's oldest medicine systems) called the Thymus Tap or Thymus Thump. As the name suggests, you tap or thump on your thymus (chest) for up to 60 seconds, several times a day. The sternum (chest bone) acts like a soundboard that vibrates and stimulates the nearby thymus gland, therefore activating T-cell production and boosting your immune system. I can't help but think of how gorillas beat their chests to show their strength... maybe they know they are boosting their immune systems too! However, when I was suffering from severe anxiety, panic attacks and PTSD, my thymus gland (left lobe specifically) became what I can only describe as frozen. I was strongly guided not to tap or thump it at all but to 'unlock' and release it with gentle downward massaging sweeps with the heel of my right hand. When my 'fight or flight' response had been triggered, I could feel, see and sense the left lobe of the gland upshift, contract and go rigid, like it had been hit with a taser. The contraction was so intense it was like my chest was being squeezed and gripped tight. The hit of stress hormones would literally shock and paralyse the left lobe, which also seemed to override anything else I tried to do, which is why it's important to perform the Thymus Gland Reset straight away.

As the thymus gland is a slightly different shape and size for everyone, the exact location may vary, but finding the tender spot can often indicate you are in the right place. When I have taught the Thymus Tap or Thymus Reset to clients, I would often guide them to slightly different areas of their chest, even some up towards their neck, close to their thyroid gland. This is in-keeping with research conducted in 2010 which scientifically proved that the thymus gland can vary in shape and size between individuals.

It also reported that the thymus gland can actually shrink with stress, but can also grow back to its original size or larger after recovery ($_5$). As I write this, my attention is taken inward to my own thymus gland, and I can intuit how it still holds trauma from the shocking experience I had during my Dark Night of the Soul. This highlights how healing is certainly a process, a peeling back of layers, which doesn't happen overnight.

As I mentioned in the 8 Step Sequence instructions, when experiencing anxiety, panic attacks or PTSD, perform the Thymus Reset (massage). During periods of depression, fatigue, lethargy, perform the Thymus Tap with all fingers and thumb together forming a beak-like shape.

Energetically, the thymus gland is also the site of the higher heart chakra which, when activated, helps us to transcend the three-dimensional reality of conditional love and access higher states of unconditional, all-encompassing, selfless and divine love and compassion. Not just towards ourselves and others, but love for the whole universe and the divine source of creation. This chakra is our connection to our true higher self where our passion and purpose come into our being. Ultimate truth and forgiveness also play a huge part in maintaining an active and open higher heart chakra, which in turn allows for a healthier immune system. Pure blissful joy is also a state that can be felt and embodied by this chakra.

Adrenal Gland Reset
If we think back to the fear/stress response, remember it all starts at the amygdala (a part of the brain), which recognises threat or danger and then relays a signal to the commander-in-chief (hypothalamus), who readies the body for action. When such an emergency occurs, the commander-in-chief is very smart and has two methods to ready and deploy her troops. Firstly via an instant message (the neurotransmitters of the central nervous system), which instructs the special-forces regiment (adrenal glands) to deploy troops immediately to fight on the front line (adrenaline and noradrenaline). This is the short term and immediate response to stress, which increases heartrate and blood pressure and dilates the lungs. The special-forces regiment (adrenaline glands), which is split into two, both of which are stationed on top of the kidneys—located very close to the psoas muscle, might I add—have within seconds mobilised and jumped into action once this message is received.

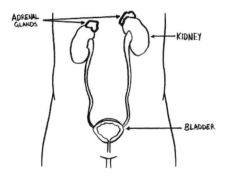

**Diagram 3. Location of the
Adrenal Glands**

The commander-in-chief then sends her second message, via the lieutenant or second-in-command (the pituitary gland), who is responsible for delivering the message personally by foot (a hormone that travels in the bloodstream to the adrenal glands). This time, instructions inform the release of the special forces back-up troops (the steroid hormone cortisol), whose job it is to offer more assistance and conduct a further recce. If the danger is still present (real or perceived, remember), they dish out energy drinks (release glucose into the blood) and if the threat is prolonged, they can even create more energy from substances they find on route (converting fat and protein into glucose). These backup troops (cortisol) also instruct the immune surveillance corps to stand down. They don't waste much time before taking R&R, which leaves the body open to other sneaky invaders (weakening the immune system). If the danger has subsided, however, the backup troops perform a clean-up and sweep, helping to regulate everything back to normal (stabilising blood pressure and reducing inflammation), allowing the initial front-line troops to return to base (adrenaline and noradrenaline are no longer released).

In physiology, this whole system is known as the hypothalamic-pituitary-adrenal (HPA) axis, and forms part of the 'fight or flight' response; however, it can become faulty. The special forces regiment can become a little too eager and overzealous to deploy troops, as is the case with prolonged stress, anxiety and panic attacks, or in worse cases, the whole system can become completely dysfunctional when the lines of command are not adhered to, as research suggests happens with PTSD. Here, the lieutenant, our secondary back-up messenger who travels on foot to the special forces regiment (adrenal glands) to conduct the clean-up, sometimes doesn't arrive or his message is not clearly understood (cortisol is not released or it doesn't do its job properly) and the special forces regiment keeps deploying more frontline troops anyway (adrenaline and noradrenaline). This constantly re-mobilises the 'fight or flight' response, which I experienced personally after my Dark Night of the Soul and PTSD. Due to my ability to gain intuitive feedback from my internal organs, I became aware of my right adrenal gland in particular becoming so hypersensitive that it would trigger and activate spontaneously. Special forces were constantly deploying even when no threat or danger was present, even when I was sat relaxing with no thoughts to trigger my 'fight or flight' response. In fact, my adrenal gland was acting like a night watchman, in a constant state of alert, primed ready for action... it actually physically tremored at the most subtle level, which reminded me of that fuzz or pulsating sensation you feel on the screen of a TV that has been left on for too long. Then, as time passed and fear subsided, my adrenal gland seemed to switch from super sensitivity to shutting down, feeling muted and unresponsive. This coincided with fatigue and grief, feelings of lethargy, depression and sadness. There are really mixed results in clinical research regarding whether this persistent activation of the 'fight or flight' response causes higher or lower cortisol levels in PTSD sufferers.

However, as more key research is conducted and more knowledge unravelled, better, scientifically proven methods for managing PSTD can be offered to those who suffer. Although we should be grateful to our commander-in-chief (hypothalamus), our lieutenant or second-in-command (pituitary gland), the various regiments (glands/organs) and troops (neurotransmitters/hormones), we can learn to override our autonomic bodily responses. Know that you can become the ultimate Major General and pull rank! By stepping in immediately and physically, we can bypass the commander-in-chief and go directly to the special forces troops and tell them to stand down! We then become our own authority and take charge of our physical body responses; however, awareness and action is needed immediately.

Using the Heel of the Hand

While performing both the Thymus and Adrenal Gland Reset, it is important to use the hand's heel, also known as the Mount of Venus in Chinese palmistry, which relates to the areas of life that the planet Venus represents in astrology. Venus, the goddess of love in Roman mythology, influences all matters of the heart—how, why and who we love, plus our most fundamental values. You may wonder what on earth this has got to do with overcoming anxiety, fear and transforming loss and grief, but Venus is concerned not only with relationships with others but, more importantly, developing a loving relationship with ourselves.

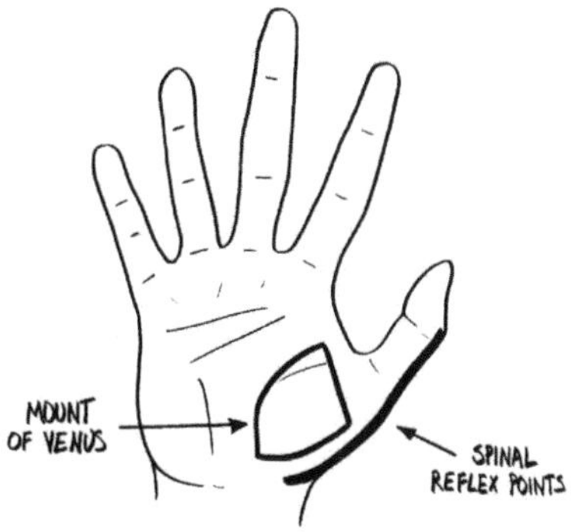

MOUNT OF VENUS

SPINAL REFLEX POINTS

Diagram 4. The Mount of Venus and Spinal Reflex Points

The edge of the thumb and heel of the hand area also reflect the spine and spinal cord, so the central nervous system in reflexology, the well-known and popular complementary therapy that studies the zones and reflex areas on the feet and hands. As the central nervous system carries incoming and outgoing messages between the brain and the rest of the body, using the Mount of Venus and the edge of the heel of the hand helps to connect our emotional heart and nervous system directly to the specific glands we are consciously resetting. In my practice as an Energy Therapist and in my reiki teaching, I have psychically seen how subtle energy can be channelled from the hands; this includes the palms and the fingers. The fingers often channel different elements—so subtle energy imbibed with fire, earth, air and water, all of which make up ether, the fifth invisible energy. Since every person is born with a particular constitution with a predominate element or elements, we can be out of balance and lacking in a particular essence. Therefore, if we use specific fingers for the reset, we could end up further destabilising an already out-of-balance constitution. Channelling fire energy where air is needed, for example. So always use the Mount of Venus and heel of the hand to be on the safe side.

Step 3 – Vagus Nerve Stimulation to Find Paradise Within
So far, we have learnt how to dissipate stress through our mighty mind-body-energy connector, the psoas muscle, how to reset our very own immune system surveillance headquarters, the thymus gland, and how to pull rank and take charge of our stress hormones via the adrenal glands. Now it's time to find paradise within with a little help from our vagus nerve, which is the longest of the 12 cranial nerves that arise directly from the brain, also known as CN X (which stands for cranial nerve 10). Although it is referred to as singular, we actually have two, a pair of vagus nerves that emerge from the right and left side of the brain in an area known as the medulla oblongata, with the right vagus nerve being more superficial, so nearer to the surface of the skin. But before you doze off, I want to explain what makes the vagus nerve so special, and

that is its long, winding nature. Vagus actually comes from the Latin word 'vagus', meaning wandering. After it exits the brain, it loops down both sides of the neck, into the chest, then into the diaphragm before finally ending up in the abdomen (see Diagram 5). Therefore, the vagus nerve has the important job of sending messages to your throat (larynx), upper chest (trachea), your heart, lungs, stomach and intestines. However, although the vagus nerve runs through most of our major organs, it does not directly innervate the thymus or the adrenal glands, which is why we needed to reset them ourselves physically in Step 2.

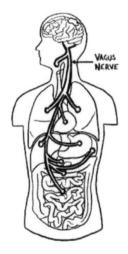

VAGUS NERVE

Diagram 5. The Vagus Nerve

But to understand the true magic of the vagus nerve and why it should become your new best friend, you need to grasp the basics of our nervous system, so with 'basic is best' in mind, let's explore that a little more. Think of your nervous system as not dissimilar to the World Wide Web, an interconnected network of nerves that carry messages to and from the brain, spinal cord and rest of your body. As you already know, the nervous system sends its messages via chemical and electrical charges called neurotransmitters and is split into two: the central nervous system (CNS), which includes your brain and spinal cord; and the peripheral nervous system (PNS), which is further broken down into three areas:

* The autonomic nervous system (ANS), which includes the sympathetic and parasympathetic functions which connect to organs and glands
* The enteric nervous system (ENS), the nerves within the gut
* The somatic nervous system (SMS), the nerves that connect to voluntary muscles

So, with the basics now covered, let's get back to the vagus nerve, which falls under the autonomic nervous system (ANS), which has the overall responsibility of regulating all the things we don't have to consciously think about like our heart rate, blood pressure and digestion. This system is further broken down into two functions: the sympathetic nervous system (SNS), which controls the already discussed 'fight or flight' response, and the parasympathetic nervous system (PSN), which controls an inbuilt system which works in opposition called the 'rest and digest' response. An easy way to remember the difference is to think about how relaxed you feel while on holiday in a *para*dise of crystal-clear blue waters and white sands—well, that's the job of the *'Para'*-sympathetic Nervous System: to relax the muscles, slow the breathing and generally make you feel stress free. So ideally, we want our autonomic nervous system to default to parasympathetic mode because, as the name suggests, 'rest and digest' stimulates healing, regeneration, relaxation and immunity, unlike 'fight or flight', which bombards our bodies with stress hormones (adrenaline, noradrenaline and cortisol) and keeps us 'wired and tired'. Over a prolonged period of time this affects our gut health too, because blood flow is diverted away from digestion, leading to decreased nutrient absorption, which eventually suppresses the immune system, leading to all-too-common inflammatory diseases like allergies, asthma, bowel disease and autoimmune disorders.

So, you might be thinking: well, not everyone is fortunate enough to have regular holidays to create that relaxation effect. But what if I told you, you don't even need a holiday to activate the parasympathetic nervous system? You can do this yourself by directly hacking into the power of the vagus nerve. There are whole programmes based around the theory of vagus nerve stimulation (VNS), one that includes the use of a pacemaker-like device implanted under the skin of the chest, a method used since the 1970s to control seizures. More recently, a study by the University of Leeds (2019) found that using a self-administered non-invasive electronic device attached to the tragus section of the outer ear for 15 minutes daily for two weeks also increased the relaxation 'rest and digest' response ($_6$). Other home-based methods to stimulate the vagus nerve include splashing your face with cold water (the diving reflex), singing or making sounds to activate the larynx, various diaphragmatic breathing techniques and the Valsalva Manoeuvre (like blowing up a balloon but with nostrils closed). However, I find the earlobe and neck technique as described in Step 3 of the 8 Step Sequence much simpler and quicker to perform!

As the instructions state, you can also add to this step by humming, singing or chanting a sound. Since the vagus nerve is a mixed nerve with both sensory and motor functions, this actually activates the vocal cords, causing vibrations that further help to stimulate the nearby vagus nerve. Any sound will do, but if you want to harness your inner chi and self-development work further, using the sound 'Om' has additional energetic benefits. The sound 'Om', which when expressed in a prolonged manner sounds like 'Aum', originates from the Sanskrit language. The meaning and interpretations of 'Om' are complex and vary according to source, but the widely accepted view is that it is the sound from which all the manifest universe emanates, so a powerful creation vibration. So be sure to think positive and relaxing thoughts while you hymn, sing or chant it! If this is something that interests you, please feel free to investigate further. As with all my self-healing and inner exploration, I have not been overly concerned with the origin of a particular belief system or technique, but more interested in what effect any practice has had on my energy, body and mind. I was intuitively guided to rub my ears and neck way before I had a conscious understanding of what I was doing, so learning to trust yourself and your gut even if it doesn't make logical sense is also part of this process.

This brings me on to another important function of the vagus nerve: its connection to the gastrointestinal tract, which consists of a mesh-like system of neurons, known as the enteric nervous system (another division of the peripheral nervous system) or what is now being called our 'second brain'. Our digestive system is not simply a dumping ground for food that gets broken down into energy or waste but an area of high sensitivity with between 200-500 million neurons lying in the walls of the oesophagus, stomach, intestines, pancreas, gall bladder and biliary tree. That's almost treble the amount in the spinal cord! So you could say that we have a gut-brain and a head-brain, and the vagus nerve is the bridge between the two, because 80% of its fibres are sensory (afferent nerves) and carry information from the body back to the brain. Therefore, how well your small intestine and large intestine muscles involuntarily contract (their motility)—so, how well your food is digested—is really down to the tone and health of your vagus nerve too. Along with our microbiome (our good and bad bacteria), it is also estimated that more than 90% of the body's serotonin, our 'happy hormone', and 50% of our dopamine, the 'pleasure and reward hormone', are also made in the gut— another reason to start feeling the love for your vagus nerve.

In terms of our energy anatomy then, the gut is also the area of the body ruled by the solar plexus chakra, the junction where the origin of the mighty psoas muscle (our super mind-body-energy connecter and bridge between our upper and lower body) and diaphragm meet. Your solar plexus chakra is your seat of willpower and where your sense of identity and your intuition is developed, not the third eye chakra, like many believe. Therefore, if you have poor gut health, not only is your immunity compromised but also your intuition. Can you see the link? Mind, body and energy are all connected!

Step 4 – Sensing for Body Awareness

Most people are aware that as human beings we have five basic senses: smell, touch, sight, hearing and taste. However, this is not technically accurate, as we do have more. The organs responsible for these senses feed information back to the brain to help us perceive our environment and the world around us. These are technically known as our exteroceptive systems: smell (olfactory system), touch (somatosensory system), sight (visual system), hearing (auditory system) and taste (gustatory system). As the name 'exteroceptive' suggests, all these systems help you to sense your external environment. The vestibular system or balance centre, located in the inner ear, is a less well-known sensing ability that helps us perceive our balance, posture and motion. When we become busy and overactive in the mind, we often disconnect from our senses. Have you ever been so preoccupied with a task that you knock yourself and, although you are aware you have done this, you don't feel the pain until later that day when you sit down to relax?

Mindfulness is the practice of becoming aware in every possible moment. Aware of our thoughts, our feelings, our behaviours and the environment around us in a non-judgemental and detached manner. Mindfulness is not just a meditation practice but a way of living, but due to our modern, fast-paced society and the need to constantly be achieving and doing, we have forgotten how to fully engage and focus on the task at hand. More so, we have forgotten how to spend time simply non-doing and being. So often it is our mind that takes us out of the present moment, catapulting us into an imaginary future. The list of endless jobs we have to do, the meetings we have to attend, even nice things like holidays and other recreational events can become stressful. Many people wish their lives away, on a non-stop merry-go-round, living for the weekend, thinking we will find peace and contentment when we achieve our next goal or reach our next destination. 'If only I could get a promotion, everything would be ok.' 'I just need to finish decorating my house, then I can relax.' Living this way, we miss the passing moments, we miss our 'now', perhaps resenting our mundane existence, which we take for granted until we have to face an unforeseen challenge or crisis. Then there's the heart, which seems to pull us back into the past, remembering times gone by, yearning and longing for a different life or to feel like we once felt. Never truly content and happy with where we are.

Sensing, then, not only brings your awareness back to the present, where you become mindful of your passing moments, immediate environment and feelings, but it also brings you deeply inward into your physical body. When we start to sense into the body in this way, with practice we can strengthen our connection to our inner state through the use of our interoceptive systems. Proprioception, for example, refers to your sense of your body position in the space around you from the receptors found in muscles and joints that send messages to the brain. Then there's thermoception, your ability to sense heat and cold; nociception, your ability to sense pain; temporal perception, the sense of passing time, to name a few. When you begin to improve your sensory abilities, you open up the mind/body connection, listening with your senses and not to your mind. In other words, your conscious mind switches off and you move away from your busy mind and thoughts, becoming more embodied, allowing room to explore your internal world more. With practice, the body will speak to you and lead you, but you have to let it become the navigational tool for your self-exploration.

Although 'Sensing' is for most highly relaxing, don't be alarmed if you experience unexpected or uncomfortable sensations in your physical body as you begin this practice, including emotions rising up. Our issues are in our tissues, and each cell of the body carries with it memory. Our body, our posture, our pain, is all a reflection of our life experiences. Therefore, the key to this practice is non-attachment to what you may sense, not following your reactions, feelings or sensations, but just witnessing them. This helps you stay grounded in the present moment, enabling you to know you are safe, safe in your environment and safe to be in your physical body, regardless of what you may be sensing internally. As you become more proficient at 'Sensing', you start to know yourself on two levels: the observing self and the experiencing self. When you get to this stage, the practice helps to build emotional intelligence and resilience, fostering deeper self-awareness.

Immediately after my Dark Night of the Soul, my body was so highly sensitised I became hyperaware of my normal physiological functions. While it is a common symptom of anxiety to feel your heart beating faster, I was constantly aware of my blood pulsing through my arteries, swirling and percolating. Initially, I didn't eat a great deal either, because the digestion process would literally blow my mind and cause me more anxiety. Due to my hyper-aroused state and growing psychic abilities, it was like being in some weird science experiment where I could actually reduce myself to a single cell. I became so small that I could travel around my digestive system, which seemed like a big scary place— so needless to say, I didn't want to eat. My physical body no longer felt a safe place for me to be, and my usual methods of meditation and 'Sensing' could no longer bring me peace because they would re-traumatise me. Whilst awake, I was in a permanent transcendental state, and my living reality felt more dreamlike than my actual dreamtime. It's like my realities switched around, and with this and the thick periods of dissociation and derealisation I was experiencing, I had to figure out another way to stabilise myself. This is when I began to continually focus and sense my feet, touching them, rubbing them and patting them with my hands to connect to them. This gave me a sense of having a physical boundary, a body, and that I was real and alive. I remember lying in my bed one afternoon and being shocked to be able to watch my husband in the kitchen, as clear as anything as if I was stood right there with him. At that point, I realised that a part of my consciousness had left my body and was in another place physically; I knew I needed to contain my energy and bring it back into my body. As crazy as this might sound, I was actually shown to use an empty toilet roll tube as a tool to help me gather myself. I visualised myself inside one and it instantly gave me a boundary, one that wasn't too dense or thick and one that I could easily penetrate if I wished. There was no top to it and no bottom so I didn't feel claustrophobic, and obviously I had to visualise a bigger-than-normal empty toilet tube to fit my whole body in. But it made me feel safer, more secure, and I was able to keep my consciousness and energy within my physical body, something I had been unable to do for weeks. It was a practice and visualisation that I came to practise regularly. As my body eased out of its frozen, hypervigilant state through the steps I describe in this book and I became more comfortable with my psychic abilities, I was able to spend more time 'Sensing' and exploring my body with its many weird sensations and feelings. Allowing myself to feel the discomfort but allowing it to pass without the panic. I am pleased to say that I can again meditate and spend extended time practising 'Sensing', both of which bring me much peace, relaxation, insight and balance.

Your personal experience of 'Sensing' will greatly depend on your level of sensitivity, anxiety, panic and the severity of any post-traumatic stress. If you are very hypervigilant, sensitised or experiencing severe PTSD, please be aware that 'Sensing' can re-traumatise. So as I previously mentioned, please begin simply by sensing your feet, knees and bottom only and pat your whole body down with your palms. Feel into this, see that the contact of your palms and skin is creating a boundary for your physical body. Although I am not sure it's for everyone, you could try my method of visualising yourself in a toilet tube... It worked for me!

Step 5 – Hara Breathing for Achieving Unification
Just as there are numerous methods of exercising our muscles (running, aerobics, weights, etc.) there are equally as many types of breathing techniques for the lungs. Prāṇāyāma, or yogic breathing, lateral thoracic breathing (which you

do in Pilates), alternate nostril breathing, 4-7-8 breathing, resonance frequency breathing (3-7 breaths per minute) to name a few. All have a different purpose and come from varying origins. In my over twenty years of teaching different exercise disciplines and meditation practices, I have tried many of them and found the greatest benefit from practising Hara Breathing. To be honest, I didn't know what I had practised for over ten years was a 'thing' until I became a Reiki Master Teacher and was conducting research while creating my training manuals. Reiki is a traditional and natural Japanese healing system, and the word *hara* simply means belly in Japanese, but is so much more than just a word. It represents an anatomical point in the physical body, an area of the body that houses our personal ki (pronounced 'key' in Japanese), and a spiritual concept meaning one's true nature. You may have heard of the more well-known terms qi or chi and tantien, used interchangeably from Eastern martial arts traditions such as tai chi, chi gong and aikido.

In reiki, Hara Breathing Technique is correctly called Joshin Kokyu Ho (*Joshin* – to focus the mind, *Kokyu* – breath/inspiration, *Ho* – method), but please know that you do not have to be reiki trained to practise Hara Breathing. What I love about this breathing technique is its three-fold positive effect: firstly, mentally, it focuses the mind; secondly, physiologically, it activates the 'rest and digest' response (parasympathetic nervous system and vagus nerve), so calms the body; and thirdly, energetically, it boosts ki. The hara is located an inch or so below the belly button (umbilicus), deep within the centre of our body towards the spine. So in its simplest form, Hara Breathing becomes a focal point on which to rest your attention, this focal point being the centre of our being (our centre of gravity). So you experience all the same benefits as you would from performing a focusing type of meditation, such as better concentration, a calmer mind and becoming more centred and present.

Physiologically then, any form of deep abdominal breathing (which forms part of Hara Breathing) is great for health as it works the diaphragm... the upside-down, dome-shaped muscle that separates the thoracic and abdominal cavities (chest and stomach). A healthy diaphragm can fully contract and flatten when we breathe in, allowing for more air to fill the lungs, and fully relax and lengthen back to its natural shape when we breathe out. Oxygen is life, and nearly every living organism on Earth needs it for survival. The average person takes approximately 20,000 breaths per day and inhales about 10,000 to 20,000 litres of air. So since we assimilate so much, you might as well learn how to do it properly! Bad posture, injury, stress, nervousness and anxiety can inhibit our breathing technique, and we end up taking small, shallower breaths where the shoulders lift and fall rather than engaging the diaphragm muscle to draw air in and out of the lungs. This then disrupts the balances of gases in the body, a reduction in carbon dioxide eventually leading to dizziness, light-headedness and the feeling of not being able to take a full breath, common symptoms that accompany a panic attack. I rarely severely hyperventilated during a panic attack, but if ever I felt light headed, I would simply cup my hands, fingers loosely together, gently rested over my mouth until the symptoms subsided. Of course, you could use a paper bag, but I am all for quickness, and this is a self-sufficient rapid response technique with minimum fuss—just make sure your hands are clean!

Deep abdominal breathing is also a pretty powerful way to 'hack' and further stimulate the vagus nerve, thus reducing heart rate, blood pressure and generally putting a break on the 'fight or flight' response. As you now know, this wandering wonder nerve runs down through the upper body and actually passes through the diaphragm muscle to reach the gut, where it innervates the smooth muscle of the gastrointestinal tract. The vagus nerve is literally listening and responding to the way we breathe and guiding our autonomic functions accordingly. So taking care of your vagus nerve and stimulating it with Hara Breathing will help you to override the physiological responses of the body we tend to think of as automatic. Therefore, we can turn off the 'fight and flight' response, and activate 'rest and digest'.

The abdomen also physically houses the following vital organs: liver, stomach, gall bladder, pancreas, small and large intestine, spleen, kidneys and adrenal glands. So when you perform Hara Breathing correctly, activating the diaphragm and your lower tummy muscle (transverse abdominis), you are also massaging your gut and internal organs (and you know now how important your gut-brain is). Even your pelvic floor gets a workout because the contents of the pelvis (bladder, sigmoid colon, womb and ovaries in women, prostate in men) are technically connected to the diaphragm via myofascial tissue... this includes your psoas muscle too.

As you probably know, any form of massage helps to improve circulation which means an increased blood flood, improved nutrient delivery and increased lymphatic fluid movement all of which are essential for a healthy immune system.

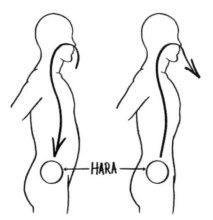

Diagram 6. Hara Breathing

Energetically, with practice and as you master Hara Breathing, you build up ki within the physical body that emanates from your aura and etheric body. You will eventually become Hara: at one with yourself and the universe rather than it simply being a location to focus on or breathing technique.

You achieve a kind of unification with everything and all that is. You are part of the universe as the universe is part of you. Just like a drop of water can be perceived as separate from its source... that is until you put that drop back in. Once the drop is returned to the ocean, it becomes unified once more, becoming one body of water, not two. The umbilicus (belly button) is also the area where as a baby we received nutrient-rich oxygen from our mothers via the umbilical cord, and energetically is the area that houses our original or pre-natal ki that we are endowed with at birth. When we cultivate a stable centre, a strong inner world, we can progress to develop other hara centres if we wish (heart and head areas). It is common to generate heat in the body while you practise Hara Breathing, and you can learn to use the increased ki to your benefit by sending it to areas of the body you may wish to heal. If you are experiencing pain or an injury, place your hands there; if you are experiencing mental anguish, send the energy through your hips, legs and feet. This will ground your energy, bringing you into your body, into the present moment and out of the conscious ego or 'monkey mind'.

If the heat becomes too much, allow your increased ki to go to any living being around you that needs extra energy, such as house plants, pets or family members. Don't force anything: it's simply just a thought and intention—where attention goes, energy flows.

Much of the New Age spiritual teaching focuses on reaching up and out, seeking higher states of consciousness, astral projection (intentionally leaving your physical body), looking for external guidance and—particularly within many religions—connection to an external force (God/Goddess/ deities). This way we tend to think of ourselves as separate from the creator or divine source and having little power. This spiritual bypassing and illusion of separation can often lead to further imbalances, a kind of top-heavy energy where our connection to the divine (crown chakra) is overemphasized and our connection to being embodied here on Earth as an individual human being (root chakra) is neglected. Much like a tree with weak roots but an abundance of leaves and foliage can easily be uprooted in storms and bad weather, a person with top-heavy energy can become easily destabilised emotionally, mentally and physically.

By practising Hara Breathing, you are learning to embody your own ki, thus your own power, which—just like the drop of water—is BOTH separate AND part of the whole ocean. You as an individual are separate in body but also part of the universal life force and essence of all that is. You become Hara when you connect to your divinity, becoming a living expression of it, instead of it simply being an external theory or concept in your mind. We are co-creators with the powerful all-being divine source, and we must hold ourselves accountable and take responsibility for our own thoughts, emotions, behaviours, actions and energy. But that is our free will; it is a choice.

It is also important to place your tongue correctly when Hara Breathing, which if you remember, is to gently rest it behind your teeth and against the roof of your mouth with jaw relaxed. Near this spot, two energy lines (meridians) come together that when stimulated can create a flowing harmonious circuit of energy within the body called the microcosmic orbit. In Traditional Chinese Medicine (TCM), the two meridians are called the Conception vessel (ren mai) and the Governing vessel (du mai). Ren mai is the major yin feminine meridian and du mai is a major yang masculine meridian. Both form just part of the sophisticated network of energy pathways that run throughout the body, and regardless of biological sex, humans have both yin and yang energies within that are constantly seeking balance. Wikipedia states that meridians do not exist as scientists have found no evidence that supports their existence. However, in 2016, researchers from Seoul National University claimed to have discovered the physical components of the Acupuncture Meridian System and named it the Primo Vascular System ($_7$), a system that is physically within the body but separate from the cardiovascular and lymphatic vessels.

So now you can see just how powerful and beneficial this simple style of breathing is, all you need to do is simply follow the instructions to perform it. No force is needed, just a gradual softening and lengthening which will come with practice, so enjoy learning to master Hara Breathing and enjoy learning to master yourself!

Step 6 – Medulla Hold for Assisting Integration
So we've looked at how anxiety and fear can affect several bodily systems such as the central nervous system, peripheral nervous system, muscular system, endocrine system and immune system, but only briefly looked at our command centre! This is where our commander-in-chief (hypothalamus) and lieutenant, our second in command (pituitary gland), are based. It's also where the medulla is located... inside the brain! The most complex organ in the human body, the brain controls all of the body's functions, much like the hard drive of a computer. Although it's mighty in function, receiving approximately 30% of the blood pumped by the heart, with information passing between neurons as fast as 250mph, it only weighs a measly 2.5-3 pounds in a human adult. Now, I'm no brain expert—it's hard enough trying to understand my own mind, let alone someone else's—so I'm going to simplify as much as I possibly can... while still being informative and hopefully interesting for you! The scientific community uses various terms to explain brain anatomy, so I will use what I feel are the simplest for the purpose of understanding why the Medulla Hold is important.

Structurally, the brain has three main parts: the cerebrum, cerebellum and the brainstem, as illustrated in diagram 7. The cerebrum is the largest part of 'grey matter', the cerebral cortex the name for that strange creased and squishy outer layer that most people picture when they think of a brain. It contains the two hemispheres: the right, controlling and processing signals from the left side of the body, and vice versa for the left hemisphere, both connected by the corpus callosum.

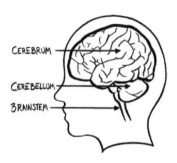

CEREBRUM
CEREBELLUM
BRAINSTEM

**Diagram 7. The Three Main
Structures of the Brain**

On each side under the creased, squishy cerebral cortex are the four lobes of the layered neocortex: the frontal lobe, the temporal lobe and the two lobes that enable you to read this book... the occipital lobe and parietal lobe. The cerebellum, or 'little brain', although connected, sits like a separate structure below and towards the back of the cerebrum, and the brainstem sits just in front, connecting the brain to the spinal cord. In terms of function then, we could say the brain has three: to receive incoming information, process this information and then to decide on an outcome/response. Unfortunately, these three functions don't neatly correlate directly to the three main structures of the brain but can be better explained in terms of our brain's purported evolution. The medulla, or more correctly termed the medulla oblongata, is a mass of neurons that relays messages between the spinal cord and cortex. It forms part of the brain stem and creates the floor of the fourth ventricle, one of the brain's cavities that are filled with cerebral spinal fluid. The medulla is responsible for keeping us alive as it controls our involuntary and automatic functions such as breathing, heart rate, body temperature, balance, and reflexes such as vomiting, coughing and swallowing.

According to neuroscientist and physician Paul MacLean (1960) in his somewhat over-simplistic Triune Brain Model ([8]), triune meaning three-in-one, he suggested that together with the cerebellum, the medulla forms the oldest and most primitive part of our brain. When these parts of our brain become activated, our 'survival state' is triggered and we act on impulse, instinct and compulsion, which is a very animalistic response. MacLean called this the 'Reptilian Brain' because he believed this part was inherited from our reptile ancestors and that the highly functioning neocortex grew over this older brain as we evolved. However, modern science now proves that even reptiles have some degree of cortex, so rather than having three separate brains in one, the human brain has modified versions of the older structures. Nevertheless, the theory is still a good one for possibly further explaining how the fear response can override conscious rational thought. If you remember, fear all stems from our amygdala, the area of the brain that perceives threat and danger which initiates the 'fight, flight or freeze' response by sending a warning signal to our commander-in-chief, the hypothalamus, who then deploys her troops. However, along with the thalamus (the relay station for all sensory information) and the hippocampus (our memory centre), both the amygdala and hypothalamus form part of another circuit of communication called the limbic system. This is a complex set of structures deep within the brain, underneath the cerebrum, which together influence our spatial awareness and our emotional state—not just fear but love, pain and pleasure too. Since our emotions are the driving force behind our behaviours, the limbic system also regulates our habitual reactions and attitudes. The amygdala attaches emotions to certain memories, and the hippocampus forges a connection between these memories and our senses before sending them away to be stored in the cortex. So when you hear a certain song that triggers a memory and emotion, or when you get a whiff of a certain perfume and it reminds you of an ex, it's these two limbic structures at work! The limbic system is also said to be related to parental behaviour and is thought to help our survival as a species, or in small communities and groups, such as connecting and bonding with others in your tribe to foster feelings of acceptance and safety. Think of a wolf pack. As a group, they cooperate and work together, therefore can protect their young, their territory and hunt more efficiently.

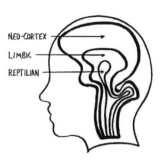

Diagram 8. Triune Brain Model

When our brain senses a threat, it is postulated that it regresses to our oldest reptilian and limbic brains, activating the 'fight, flight or freeze' response, helping to keep us safe. This survival state is needed for physical danger but can cause issues when the threat becomes more emotional in nature. For example, losing a job (your identity, purpose and financial security), isolation (lack of nurturing support) and loss of a loved one (abandonment) can all trigger the limbic system to feel threatened. Remember that's the part of the brain that evolved to keep the tribe safe where social interaction, having a role or responsibility, attachment and nurturing support forms the basis of safety. With certain anxiety disorders and with trauma, the brain can actually become stuck in the more reptilian and limbic function, so in 'survival and emotional state'. Although we might know a certain emotional response and behaviour is not helpful, it's not enough to stop the reptilian brain and limbic systems from activating. Unlike the neocortex—'neo' meaning new— which is the most highly evolved part of the brain, allowing us to think rationally, have conscious thought, reason, plan, analyse, problem solve and make decisions about the future, the older part of the brain doesn't register the concept of logic or time, which is why fears from the past can affect us in the present.

The physical contact and warm soothing touch of your palms placed directly on the back of the skull (occipital bone), where the more instinctual part of the brain is located, can calm this survival response. This will bring back balance to the physical body, which will then lead to calmer emotions (control of our limbic system) and clearer thinking (better use of our neocortex). Remember, once the fear response is activated, positive affirmations only go so far. Resetting the physical body should take priority to regain homeostasis, then we can better explore and reprogram our emotional response (limbic system) through collaboration with our logical neocortex to rewire our pattern of thoughts and beliefs.

Energetically, we have a lesser-known chakra located at the back of the head and neck; it is of a diagonal alignment from the nape of the neck up into the occipital area (that's the bony back of the skull). It's named the medulla chakra because it is an energy entry point that connects directly to the medulla oblongata. Just as our digestive system assimilates the food we eat, this chakra absorbs external life force before transforming it into our own ki. It then directs this energy up to the crown chakra, where it gets distributed throughout the rest of the etheric body. However, this chakra began an upgrade, for want of a better term, from 2016 onwards. This upgrade was needed because the incoming life force energy we were being asked to assimilate was from outside of our solar system. I know this sounds wacky, but hear me out... We live on Earth, and the Earth is part of our solar system, which revolves around our star, the Sun. Any energy and cosmic radiation that enters Earth's atmosphere also influences us as humans since we are bioelectrical beings. For example, light and heat produced by solar nuclear fusion travel to Earth as photons, and this is what makes it possible for life to exist. Trees need sunlight to grow and we need the oxygen that they produce to breathe. Physically, we need the Sun so our body can make Vitamin D to keep our bones, teeth and muscles healthy. Our Sun and the rest of our solar system orbits the centre of the Milky Way galaxy... a supermassive black hole called the Galactic Centre, also known as Sagittarius A. Our Milky Way galaxy, along with several hundred other galaxies, are contained within the Local Virgo Supercluster. Then, beyond that, the Laniakea Supercluster (pronounced Lan-e-a-kay-a) which cosmologists defined in 2014 as 'a huge cosmic web'. If you haven't seen it yet, you definitely should (₉). *Laniakea* is Hawaiian for 'immeasurable heaven/sky', and it is certainly that. If you ask me… it looks a lot like a human nervous system of epic proportion!

Well, our galaxy entered a new region of the cosmos, and the external life force energy our bodies are now being asked to assimilate is unlike anything humans have needed to integrate before. This led to a backlog and build-up of energy, just like how a pipe becomes blocked if excess debris accumulates. Many people, albeit unknowingly, had and still have difficulties with its upgrade, causing a whole host of physical symptoms such as neck ache, sore throats, trouble sleeping and heaviness in the sinus and eyes. I must add here that I'm not sure if cosmologists have scientific proof of our solar system entering a new part of the cosmos… yet. This is what I intuit and my spiritual team tells me.

Just as the digestive system can struggle to break down certain foods, the old medulla chakra found it difficult to assimilate the new incoming energy, hence its upgrade. Interestingly, I have been guided by an Archangel named Metatron to call this the Medulla Integration Point moving forwards, rather than a chakra, due to old and ancient teachings also needing to evolve just as we are. When there is a build-up of cosmic energy at the Medulla Integration Point, and with extreme anxiety, panic and trauma, our older chakras can become overwhelmed, in particular the nearby third eye and crown chakras. This excess build-up and overwhelm of energy causes a rapid spinning and speeding up of the microcosmic orbit, which if you remember from the Hara Breathing explanation is the flow of the main feminine and masculine energy meridians, Ren mai and du mai in Traditional Chinese Medicine (TCM). This can also affect the pulse rate of the cerebrospinal fluid (CSF), since at one end the medulla has direct access to its production and circulation via the fourth ventricle, and at the other end it narrows to become the central canal of the spinal cord. If you are familiar with yoga concepts, the Sushumna Nadi or main energy pathway of the body is accessed here.

By placing your hands in what I call the Medulla Hold, you are helping to regulate the cerebrospinal fluid pulse but also helping to offset and release any backup of cosmic energy at the Medulla Integration Point. This will help your etheric body better assimilate life force energy, in turn balancing the third eye chakra and crown. This ultimately reduces pressure on and in the brain, its glands, structures and nerve cells, including the limbic system, allowing it to function as a coherent whole and not as three separate regions.

Step 7 – Crystalline Matrix Alignment to Strengthen a New Foundation
Up until this point I have been able to validate the use and purpose of each of the steps with a little scientific backing, but this section will need you to adopt an open mind, to be receptive to a possibility that may oppose your point of view and/or beliefs. You don't have to agree, or argue for or against for that matter, just remain open. So without further ado...

The crystalline matrix is a network and web of light vibration connected to your light body, which is both the foundation of your subtle energy field and the vehicle for your soul/spirit to access other dimensions. Most people can picture a two-dimensional shape, which looks flat and static; even a three-dimensional shape, which adds depth where it begins to occupy physical space. However, beyond that, dimensions get a little harder to visualise and perceive, especially via words only, so that's where things will get a little tricky, because the crystalline matrix, although two-dimensional, merges into our fifth-dimensional and beyond light body! I can now hear people starting to hum the opening theme tune to *The Twilight Zone*, but just before you write this whole thing off... to get a truly better understanding of this concept, we need to start back at what we already know.

If we start with the physical body, we have several well-known physiological systems that keep our body functioning: the reproductive system, urinary system, integumentary (skin/nails) system, lymphatic system, respiratory system, cardiovascular system, skeletal system, myofascial system, muscular system, immune system, digestive system, limbic system, nervous system and endocrine system. The heart is responsible for pumping blood through the blood vessels (veins, arteries and capillaries), which together form the cardiovascular system. The lungs are responsible for gaseous exchange and respiration, which form the respiratory system. However, although separate in terms of their purpose, they are also interconnected and work very closely together. For example, the respiratory system relies on the cardiovascular system to deliver the oxygen it has gathered, so they interact and depend on each other to fulfil their functions.

Energetically, we also have many systems with specific functions that could be seen as separate but are really interconnected, the main difference being... most people can't see them. This whole topic is huge and certainly not within the scope of this book to discuss, so I am going to give a quick overview.

What I call our 'Subtle Energy Anatomy' is not a new concept but has been around for over 3500 years within traditional Eastern medicine. Widely accepted practices such as acupuncture, acupressure, herbal remedies, cupping and various massage therapies all seek to keep the body's subtle energy systems flowing. What tends to confuse people the most regarding 'Subtle Energy Anatomy', however, is use of the terms qi/chi, ki and prana or 'universal life force energy'. These are certainly the most common and are sometimes used interchangeably, but really differentiate between where a particular concept and teaching originated. Qi or chi is of Chinese origin, ki of Japanese origin and prana of Indian origin, but these aren't the only names that you might come across; there are many other terms that refer to the vital energy that flows through every living being.

In Traditional Chinese Medicine, qi/chi is further broken down into different essences once inside the body. The best way I can explain this is... Water is a clear fluid until you add a flavoured cordial, then it becomes a different type of water but fundamentally still fluid. So, kundalini, nutritional chi, prenatal chi, protective chi and pectoral chi are all chi...

but you could say a different flavour with a slightly different function. However, this more detailed understanding isn't needed for this book. Much like our veins and arteries carry blood, meridians are pathways or channels for our chi to flow within the physical body and the lower dantian, a storage place for the chi, just as the gall bladder is a storage place for bile. When practising Hara Breathing, which is of Japanese origin, we focus our attention to the lower hara, which is a storage place for ki, and I believe that although they have different names, both are the same in function. The other two hara centres are at the heart centre (middle dantian) and head centre (upper dantian), both organs which produce powerful electromagnetic fields. Recent research by Heart Math Institute (2015) has stated that the heart generates the most powerful electromagnetic field of any of the body's organs, sixty times greater in strength than the field generated by the brain ([10]).

If we look at the ancient practice of yoga, which originated in India over 5000 years ago, it isn't simply a form of exercise as most people think but rather a system to harness prana to attain self-realisation by transcending body and mind to achieve union with the divine. Specific postures (asana), the use of breathing techniques and connecting and directing energy to the chakra system help merge our outer- and inner-self, mind and body, physical self with non-physical self.

In Sanskrit, chakra can be translated as 'wheel', and these wheel-like vortexes are very different from the hara/dantien in that they draw energy into the body and emanate energy as opposed to being like storage sites. The seven best-known chakras are the crown, third eye, throat, heart, solar plexus, sacral and root. These chakras, although connected to the physical body, are actually located in the auric layers of your energy field. I've spoken in more detail of a few chakras already, namely the root chakra regarding the psoas/fear connection, the higher heart chakra for the thymus/immune connection, the solar plexus for the vagus nerve/intuition connection and the medulla integration point regarding the brain/cosmic energy integration. We do have many more chakras, such as the minor chakras at each joint and lesser-known major chakras such as the earth star, gaia gateway, soul star, stellar gateway, universal gateway, etc., with each connecting to another outer auric layer and energy body. Think of how those Russian dolls fit inside each other: the first inner doll, the smallest, would be the physical body, and each larger doll an expanded and ascended layer of our being. However, the layers are not separate like the dolls are; each of our energy bodies can collapse into and expand out of the preceding or proceeding layer. These layers can sometimes be seen within the energy field or aura of a person too. Now, most people have probably heard someone say 'they have a great aura about them' or 'they had a great presence'. Many people are referring to this very phenomenon, even if they can't explain or fully quantify with words what they mean by such a statement. It is the energy, thus frequency and vibration, that the person is emanating which is being felt for most on a very unconscious level. Just like the visible light spectrum, all frequencies have a particular wavelength and colour. A technique called 'Kirlian Photography', invented by an electrician named Seyyon Davidovitch Kirlian in 1939, purportedly catches such colours of living beings, but my scientific head is a little sceptical, although such a technique does make for some truly magnificent art that catches the electromagnetic discharge of an object or person. If you haven't seen such photos, check them out! There are many other patterns and flows within our energetic anatomy too, but I have only discussed the most common and the most relevant for this book.

So now we come to an energy layer which is not so traditional but has always existed. Many people are now able to feel, perceive and know that their energy layers and energy bodies extend beyond what the ancient Eastern teachings have taught us.

But to make the invisible (to most) at least remotely perceivable, I am going discuss crystals so you may better understand the nature of the Crystalline Matrix of the human body. However, please bear with me, because making something non-physical physical is no easy feat!

You may have thought that crystal lovers such as myself are nuts when we speak of charging our 'precious' in the moonlight or when people carry them to keep away the bad juju, but let me explain how they work! A crystal—or more accurately termed, a 'crystalline solid'—can only be classified as such if it has a highly organised microscopic structure, meaning all its atoms are positioned in accurate distances and angles from one another. The 'crystal lattice' is the name given to this symmetrically ordered pattern that continually repeats itself, spreading out in all three dimensions. So sugar, sand, salt and snowflakes are all technically crystals because they have a crystalline lattice, whereas glass is not because it has no ordered internal structure. However, regular beach sand and salt differ from sugar and snowflakes because they are considered minerals. Minerals not only have a crystalline lattice but must also consist of an inorganic compound. Sand mainly consists of silicon dioxide (SiO_2), more commonly known as quartz, and salt mainly consists of the inorganic compound sodium chloride ($NaCl$). Sugar, on the other hand, is organic, so is a crystal but can't be considered a mineral. Knowing such interesting facts... Will you ever look at your sugar and salt the same again, I wonder?! But let's keep on track. If I lost you back there, in simple terms... all minerals are crystals, but not all crystals can be classified as minerals, and should the crystal structure change, the result would be a different mineral. The internal structure (crystal lattice) together with its chemical composition is what gives minerals and crystals their healing properties. Their beautiful colours, facets and geometric shapes that are so aesthetically pleasing to the eye are a direct result of their internal structure and chemical composition. Crystals develop from gas or liquid because only in such fluid states are their atoms free to bond together into such an ordered manner... creating their crystalline lattice. However, as is the case with quartz, sometimes the crystalline lattice is not exactly symmetrical, perhaps an extra atom crams in or a slighter bigger atom, but their electrical charge always remains balanced.

When any energy is put into quartz-based crystals in the form of pressure, heat or light, you displace the atoms upsetting the negative and positive balance causing an electrical charge to appear. This is known as piezoelectricity, and I would bet that you've had first-hand experience of such a phenomenon! The battery in a quartz watch causes the mineral to regularly expand, creating a pulse which is how it keeps time. An ultrasound machine used to scan the body uses quartz to attain the high-frequency soundwaves needed to create that picture of your insides appear on the screen. In fact, quartz is a common component found in many modern technological devices such as mobile phones, television receivers and even spacecraft. Most of the solid material you see around you is in fact crystalline, and its study has given rise to some pretty amazing discoveries! If you are interested in learning more about this topic, 'Cristales; A world to discover' is a teaching and outreach exhibit created in celebration of the United Nations 2014 'International Year of Crystallography' and is a great resource [11].

So let's bring this back... Much like a crystal has an internal crystalline lattice, the human body could also be said to be crystalline, most certainly on the astral planes, but even on a smaller scale at the physical level. Perhaps you've been unfortunate enough to have developed gallstones whereby excess cholesterol (a fatty substance in your blood) forms into tiny solid crystalline forms, causing pain and discomfort. Gallstones should more accurately be called gall crystals, in my opinion... although that makes them sound pleasant! Then there's human bone and tooth enamel, which consist of a mineral called hydroxyapatite, which grows in hexagonal crystals. Recent research in 2018 found that a fractal-like hierarchical organisation of bone actually begins at the nanoscale, which contributes to the structural integrity of bone [12]. As I write this, I am shown the famous 'Vitruvian Man' by artist Leonardo da Vinci, reminding me to mention that geometry (points, lines, shapes and space) forms the fundamental template for all of life in the universe. Our 'Subtle Energy Anatomy' is no different, and one particular aspect known as our light body is like a multidimensional geometric sphere and the crystalline matrix its foundational structure. And to quote Yoda from *Star Wars*: 'Luminous beings we are, not this crude matter.' I couldn't agree more, because we are multidimensional beings not just a physical body. I did ask Archangel Metatron, whose area of expertise is Sacred Geometry—it's definitely not mine, because I'm rubbish at maths—why it's called the human Crystalline Matrix and not a crystalline lattice like in a crystal, and his answer was this.

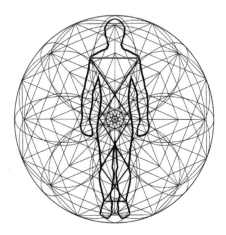

Diagram 9. The Crystalline Matrix

'The crystalline matrix of the human body is the two-dimensional grid of codes and geometry which the three-dimensional human energy lattice expands from, eventually leading to the fifth-dimensional and beyond light body... the evolved light human who can travel between dimensions.' Diagram 9 is a very crude interpretation of the human crystalline matrix with expanding human lattice, and although I was unhappy with my very basic illustration attempt, I was guided to include it to help people vaguely perceive our beautiful geometric light form.

In summary then, your chakras, your auric layers, your subtle energy bodies, already exist, including your light body, even if you are not consciously accessing them at this time. You see, dimensions are not some physical place that you arrive at, but frequency states that you access from within. You could say that humans are evolving from Homo sapiens to Homo luminous, developing the ability to perceive the physical world and universe as it really is... light, vibration and frequency. Also, for those who are more abreast of spiritual concepts, you may have heard of the term Merkaba (a two-star tetrahedron), which is a rather outdated concept due to the speed at which human transformation is taking place. Due to humanity undergoing a mass spiritual awakening, some people are having certain energy layers spontaneously activate even if they are unaware and not actively seeking such transformation. Practising the Crystalline Matrix Alignment hand positions will help integrate the light body foundation into the physical body (which if you notice are on major joints) and will also help stabilise the light body should an activation occur. We are moving away from a time of healing our parts, fragments and less evolved energy anatomy, to healing through the whole, in completeness, as we truly are.

The chakras and other energy layers actually disperse when the light body is accessed, which is often in transient spurts when consciousness is fifth dimensional and beyond. Practising the Crystalline Matrix Alignment also has physical benefits, because such criss-crossing movements of the hands help to build connections between the right and left side of the brain (the job of the corpus callosum), which means new neural pathways can more easily form, allowing information to pass more freely between the two hemispheres of the brain. Again... we are moving away from polarised separation and becoming whole beings.

Step 8 – Figure 8 Pose to Lock It In!
Human bioenergetics, a field of biochemistry, is the scientific study of how energy flows between cells and tissues in organisms. Now, we are not talking about subtle energies here, such as chi, ki and prana, but the study of different cellular and metabolic processes that influence energy production and utilisation within the cells of the body. Thousands of biochemical, bioelectrical and biomagnetic

reactions take place within these cells every single second. The mitochondria, the fundamental structure within nearly every cell of your body, converts energy from the foods we eat into adenosine triphosphate (ATP), the essential energy molecule. Mitochondria are the powerhouse of the human cell, because without ATP, cells would start to die, and eventually the whole organism would die too.

Over the last hundred years or so, a multidisciplinary team of scientists, philosophers and conventional physicians have all contributed towards evidence-based bioregulatory medicine or BioMed for short. Such practices focus more on the cause than the symptom, aim to treat the individual and not the disorder, and use non-toxic treatments instead of pharmaceutical means. It's basically the science behind the ancient wisdom and ways of natural healing that have also utilised developments in technology. Therapies and devices within the BioMed field are growing rapidly... transcutaneous electrical nerve stimulation (TENS), bioenergetic analysis, polarity therapy, energy medicine, homeopathy, kinesiology, heart rate variability (HRV), muscle testing, etc. All of which are underpinned by the notion that the body has an energy field that exhibits three states: a positive outflowing state, a negative inflowing or receptive state, and a neutral state.

Pretty much like how a single atom, the basic building block of matter, has positively charged protons, negatively charged electrons and neutral neutrons. Although ancient hands-on healing practices have been around for centuries, healing modalities such as reiki, massage, craniosacral therapy, shiatsu, cupping, Thought Field Therapy (TFT), faith healing, religious prayer healing, etc. are only now starting to be taken seriously in terms of their health-promoting benefits in the scientific community. In fact, such methods of hands-on healing have even been given a new name and are all grouped under the branch of Biofield Therapy.

A key player in this area was Dr Wilhelm Reich (1897-1957), who coined the term 'Orgone Energy' and was a psychoanalyst and Austrian doctor way ahead of his time who lived a very interesting and colourful life. His out-of-the-box thinking and ideas regarding healing the human body eventually saw him imprisoned and several of his books burnt and banned in America. It's Reich who we have to thank for the current rise and popularity in 'Orgonite' pieces, which are a combination of tiny crystals and various metal shavings in resin most commonly formed in the shape of a pyramid. Personally, I've never used such pieces because I prefer to know exactly what mineral or metal I am energetically working with. Reinhold Voll (1909-1989), another mastermind behind the development of BioMed, was a German physician and engineer who in the 1940s discovered that electrical conductivity on the skin varied in relation to location and that the most conductive points corresponded to the known acupuncture points lying along meridians from Traditional Chinese Medicine. He then went on to develop electro-acupuncture according to Voll (EAV) machines and electrical conductivity metering (ECM). Today, however, less cumbersome equipment is used, and you can purchase nifty little pens that emit an electrical charge and can be used to stimulate acupuncture points!

Wayne Cook (1910-1985) had many professions, but it wasn't until he had the opportunity to run an abandoned mineral mine that he discovered the electrochemical, biomagnetic and psychoenergic flows of the human body ($_{12}$). From his intensive research, he discovered that the reason water dowsing is possible (an ancient divination method of detecting underground water with the use of a dowsing rod) is due to the electrical energy force within the mineral water pulling the rod. His research then led him to discover that for both men and women, positively charged energy enters from the left side of the body and exits as negatively charged energy through the right. Since the hands and feet follow this pattern too, holding your hands and feet in certain positions can bring harmony but also reverse biomagnetic polarity. One such well-known position has been referred to as 'Cook's Hook Up' in honour of Wayne, which when performed brings the polarity of the body back into balance, unscrambling the mind and calming the emotions. Even before my mental illness, as a means of personal energetic self-care I would often perform an adapted version of this position, which I named the 'Figure 8 Pose' because when I did it I would see flowing energies in my body doing the shape of a figure eight. For example, a figure-eight flow in the legs (right ankle to left knee, to right hip, to left hip, down to right knee, to left ankle) or the whole body (from right ankle to groin, to opposite shoulder). Not only did this 'Figure 8 Pose' help to balance the polarity of my body, but it also gave me a sense of containment and protection, helping to stabilise an expansive energy field. If you draw the number '8', you will feel how the movement is flowing, contained and eternal. Over time as I did this, I began to see not only the larger figure-eight flows of energy but smaller figure-eight flows too, right down to my DNA (short for deoxyribonucleic acid) where my genetic coding resides. The 'Figure 8 Pose' is so simple and inconspicuous it can literally be performed anytime and in any setting. I used to often adopt the position while in meetings at work or if I could feel my energy was being drained by another. I would also end any self-healing practices with this pose and then the 8 Step Sequence as it developed, because I was shown how it acts as a seal or container, creating a 'locking in' effect that would hold my now more stabilised body, mind, emotions and subtle energies in place for longer.

You may have noticed that I also gave an alternative end position to the 8 Step Sequence, which I call the Mastering Me Loop. Being an Earth Empath means you are more sensitive to changes that happen to planet Earth, such as magnetic field disturbances, earthquakes, fires and superstorms, etc. Some but not all Earth Empaths also become more attuned to changes taking place on other planets too... solar flares and solar wind from the Sun, moon phases and other planetary retrogrades (where planets appear to change direction from the perspective of Earth). Having PTSD symptoms (hyperarousal and extreme sensitivity to any stimulus) along with such abilities was too much for me to handle, so I was guided for a short time to disconnect my energy from the Earth's magnetic field. To do this I had to isolate my own energy and find stability from within and not from the Earth itself as we are commonly guided to do. I include this position here in case any Earth Empaths who read this would benefit from reducing any overwhelming sensations and symptoms due to their unique sensitivity. I simply placed the soles of my feet together, allowing my knees to fall open into a diamond shape, and placed my hands together in a prayer/namaste position (gassho in Japanese), creating a closed, looping circuit of energy. Please note there was nothing religious about my hand position but a linking of polarities, negative to positive charge but contained within myself. I used the Mastering Me Loop for only a few months until I was stable enough mentally and physically to open up my energy to the Earth's magnetic influences again. Since that time, I've mostly used the 'Figure 8 Pose' but do on occasion, when I feel called to, use the Mastering Me Loop as well. I will add... most people are deprived and deficient in their connection to Earth energy, and most extremely sensitive Earth Empaths have probably already discovered their own way of managing their abilities. Therefore, please use your own discernment as to which end pose you should finish your 8 Step Sequence with.

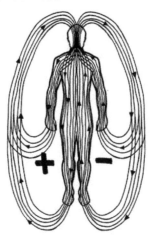

Diagram 10. Body Polarity

PART 2:

Transforming Loss and Grief

CHAPTER 7

My Understanding of Loss and Grief

Shedding a Light

It was Angel Ezekiel (pronounced e-ze-key-el) who really shed a light on my understanding of loss and grief. I will be quite frank here, I shit myself the first time his energy came forth, because he announced his arrival with, 'I'm the angel of death.' My conscious mind went into panic mode; I pleaded with him, telling him I was scared and wasn't ready to die. But then I realised my body wasn't following suit, and when I actually checked in with my gut feeling and intuition, I knew he wasn't about to take me. I guess on reflection it wasn't his energy that seemed frightening but my own perception of his words. At this point I had communicated and worked with plenty of angelic beings before; they would often show up when I was performing an energy healing on myself or another. They would assist me if I allowed, relay divine guidance and messages that I could pass on, but they always appeared as lights to me, huge beings of light varying in colours, frequency and vibration who would telepathically communicate. Angel Ezekiel, however, sounded and looked different, he felt more man than angel and spoke through his mouth with words, but as always, I trusted my intuition and I felt no threat, just divine presence. So I remained open.

He spoke... 'It's not death you fear but the realm of the underworld.' My disbelieving mind abruptly repeated back,

'Underworld?! WTF!?', not actually talking to him but to myself. Memories of the film *Thor* and the nine realms flooded my mind, wondering if it contained subliminal mind-control messages that were now playing out. Or was I just simply making this up? My logical mind and ego had always had my back, like an internal verifier I guess, checking the reliability and validity of what I heard, like a good scientist trying to prove myself wrong, but this time it was more a hindrance, trying to block the incoming message.

Then he cleared his throat, as if to interrupt my internal dialogue and debate to get my attention... 'You have already experienced death, a complete death of the ego during your Dark Night of the Soul, but also when you experience your light body. This closely resembles life without a physical body, so physical death to you.' I paused, contemplating his words, sensing into them, realising there was truth in what he had said, feeling more lightness than heaviness. I postulated, 'So, ok, if I don't fear death, what is the underworld and why do I fear that?'

His response: 'The underworld is a dark place of deepest fear, hurt and pain, a place of lost souls.' I shuddered as I began hearing the cries and screams and feeling the darkness coming from there, so I quickly changed tack.

'What do you want?' I said abruptly, feeling fear again.

'You have asked for help, you have asked to be shown how to heal your anguish, and I am here to assist. Conduct a Life Review and free yourself from your pain. Release your grief and you will transform.' Then his energy pulled back.

About three months after my Dark Night of the Soul, my panic attacks began subsiding and my hypervigilant and sensitised body and mind started becoming numb. My symptoms seemed to gradually change from being on constant high alert to feeling myself sinking into strange periods of profound disorientation and fog where my body felt like it was turning off. Yes, I experienced dissociation and depersonalisation which would trigger panic, but for the most part, I felt like a thick dark cloud had descended over me. My world felt so grey, there seemed to be no colour or life anywhere I looked, then that grey eventually became black. All I felt was vast emptiness and darkness, a deep, deep sadness where I was void of anything but sorrow and anguish. I began to wonder whether I was now experiencing depression, but in my heart, I knew it was something else. I understood on a mental level that depression was caused by chemical imbalances in the brain, and I guess I had always perceived it as a state of apathy where you don't have the will or desire to do anything and feel helpless. Although I did feel hopeless, I did have help from my spiritual team and the desire and will to heal myself, knowing that on some level I was supposed to be experiencing such feelings, so I didn't consider myself depressed. Every time I asked my guides and the angelic realm for guidance, I was repeatedly shown that I needed to focus on 'grief work'. At first, I vaguely thought I understood; it made sense to my mind, as I had lost my Nanny Cath a few months before the onset of my mental illness. So I proceeded to process all my emotions connected to her and how she'd passed. Another two months went by, but over and over again, I was told 'grief work' at every self-healing. I started to question my guidance because I truly believed and felt that I no longer held grief where my Nan was concerned. She was lucky, I guess. She was 92 years old when she passed and hadn't suffered towards the end of her life; she literally just collapsed one day and stopped breathing. So it wasn't a painful and traumatic experience like many people have to endure, which I was grateful for, so I couldn't understand why I still found it so difficult to move through the grief I was feeling.

Much to my frustration, the message and guidance didn't change, and eventually, I toyed with the idea that I might be missing something vital. I was faced with the prospect that my idea and perception of what grief actually was might not be totally accurate or complete. So I decided to forget everything I thought I knew about grief, unlearning and letting go of what I had perceived as my truth, and started again. I quickly came to discover that grief is simply the emotional response to loss, so when Angel Ezekiel eventually made his debut appearance and told me to conduct a Life Review, I instantly put two and two together. I needed to review my entire life and make note of any events that may have resulted in some form of loss. This new understanding opened up a whole new possibility for my healing and gave me some leverage with which to work, where I had, until then, felt like I kept hitting a dead end. Where I had felt stuck and resigned to the fact that I would remain trapped in that weird state of inertia forever, I now had hope and a new direction to follow. I came to understand that any form of loss actually comes from experiencing some form of change. Just re-read that sentence, then read it again!

This was my biggest revelation—a simple one, but huge nonetheless. It was like a light bulb blasted on, a dinging bell, a complete shift in my perception, neuroplasticity in action! My new truth had been discovered: 'If the emotions of grief come from loss and loss can come from change, loss and grief are inevitable because life is always changing.' This new concept blew my mind. It was so simple—and yet why hadn't I recognised it before? Well, perhaps I had recognised it on a purely mental level, but I had not truly felt it. My mind quickly shifted from amazement to curiosity then to feeling slightly annoyed. Why wasn't I taught this simple fact before? Why wasn't I prepared for how to deal with loss and grief in school? Why is the topic of loss and grief so awkward and uncomfortable for so many, and why do most people shy away from it even when it's the one certainty in life?

Reflecting on my new-found truth, I began to see all the ways in which life changes and so all the ways we can potentially experience loss. From the most fundamental changes such as the days of the week, the weather, the seasons, to more complex changes such as biological aging and the choices we make every single day that eventually map out our life, all of which are completely natural. But I felt a shift within, from linear thinking where there is a start, middle and an end, to seeing life as a continual process of transition and transformation: birth, growth, then decay, repeated over. From the smallest scale of each passing moment to the largest scale... a whole human life. On top of this continual process of transformation of birth and death, we layer our existence with labels and identities. We acquire new roles—we become a new friend, a sister, a mother, a brother, a father, a grandparent. We become a student, an apprentice, a musician, a dancer, a doctor, a manager or teacher (otherwise known as ego structures). We label ourselves, putting us into tiny neat little boxes, all of which build to create our sense of self and identity—even our purpose in life and who we think we are. We take on different roles and even behave in certain ways to fit each of our identities. This falsely creates a sense of safety in certainty and predictability. I cringe when I hear stereotypical comments such as 'Don't you change, girl; don't you change for no man', or when a man proclaims, 'I'm not changing for you. This is who I am, take me or leave me.' While I am all for empowerment and creating strong, healthy boundaries, it is naïve and limiting to avoid growth and change. Healthy relationships need transformation to exist. The only guarantee and constant in this life IS change, it is not possible to remain the same... change will always come. For some, it will come easily and for others, like me (I am a Taurus Sun... a fixed Earth sign after all), it will prove more difficult. When I bought my first home, I was no longer the daughter who relied on her parents to put a roof over her head. When I got married, I was no longer the single and spontaneous adrenaline junkie who could just up and travel, seeking the next big adventure. After graduating I was no longer the carefree student, but a young adult starting to pave a career with new responsibilities. After my mental illness and leaving my fifteen-year university career, I was no longer 'sporty Emma'. I mean, I didn't even know what clothes to wear. I had lived in trainers and shorts pretty much my whole adult life, and without this, I didn't know who I was any longer. For every change experienced, I had to evolve and grow, becoming a different version of myself, which meant losing the version beforehand. That was my second revelation, learning that I was grieving myself. My old self was dying but my new self was yet to be born. I was in that weird, liminal 'bardo' state, not only in-between dimensions of existence energetically and spiritually, but physically in-between who I was and who I was becoming. My fear of death and dying (or so I thought) was so profound that an eerie feeling of unease and anxiety would come over me every time I experienced an ending—the end of a film, when I finished a task I was focused on, when there was a change to my immediate environment, and even at the end of the day... which sounds insane, I know, but let me explain. As daytime becomes dusk, there is a transition. Physically, light diminishes as darkness unfolds, but there are also changes in the atmosphere during these transitional periods. Being an Earth Empath, I would literally feel the death of the day, which is why I would fight off a panic attack just as the light would begin to diminish. Seasonal shifts such as spring to summer happen gradually so they are not felt so intensely, although as I type this, I am reminded that my PTSD occurred in December, the onset of the densest seasonal shift... winter. But going back to the 24-hour cycle, there are actually four magnetic seasons to a single day: morning is akin to spring, noon akin to summer, early evening akin to autumn, and night akin to winter. If you are a HSP, an Earth or Molecular Empath, you may experience strange sensations and feelings at these transitional times of the day due to changes in the Earth's electromagnetic field, atmospheric pressure and ionisation of the air. Most people don't have conscious awareness of such changes, so their mind creates its own stories and reasons for their strange feelings, which adds further complications in understanding their mental and emotional state.

I didn't know it then, but I was being initiated into the very ancient and misunderstood darker realms of the divine feminine energy, the powerful portal between life and death, the doorway between this life and the next. I had to get comfortable with being at the crossroads and feeling this dying process so tangibly to be able to fully claim my ability as a death doula, a woman who serves as a guide to souls who are physically dying. Only, I don't need to be physically at someone's side to help their energy and consciousness leave their body. I can assist them in letting go of their attachments to the physical world and Earthly plane remotely, from a distance. In many religions, the name 'psychopomp' is given to the ones who guide souls into the afterlife. However, many people also require similar assistance in transforming their energy and emotional state while still living and in the physical body here on Earth. So, I eventually came to see my job as being the same for the living, the dying, and in some cases the dead… which is helping people transform energetically. I was always going to be limited with how many people I could work with directly, so I will share how you can transform your own emotional energy in Chapter 11, but first you must take a deeper look into your own loss and grief. That means first having a clear concept of the terminology involved.

Terminology
When I began exploring loss and grief more deeply, I soon found myself frustrated because a lot of different words and terms seemed to be used to explain the same thing. Loss, grief, mourning and bereavement were terms used interchangeably, but I came to understand that they do mean different things. 'Bereavement' and 'mourning' are most commonly used when we speak of death and the passing of another. The bereaved is someone who is deprived of another's presence through death. Mourning is the term used to describe a period whereby a person's death is expressed in a more outwardly directed manner by the bereaved. When a person is 'in mourning', they may exhibit particular behaviours such as wearing black, organising the funeral, withdrawing from social events and acting respectfully. Flying a flag at half-mast is a respectful way of honouring the passing of someone important, or a

significant event such as Memorial Day or other National Days of Remembrance. The length of mourning is highly individual and is often influenced by cultural customs, rituals and religious beliefs. In Western culture although many people start mourning immediately following the death of a loved one, or in some cases even before, they often begin their more official mourning period the day of the funeral and wake when they say their goodbyes to the physical aspect of the person who has died. 'Loss' and 'grief' are also terms commonly used when we talk about the death of another, but unlike 'bereavement' and 'mourning', they also refer to other life experiences, which we shall explore next in more detail. These interpretations will not fit everyone's experience and that is ok, but I want to at least highlight some distinctions between them before we dive deeper into the process of transforming loss and grief.

CHAPTER 8

Understanding Your Loss

What is Loss?

Loss is technically the end or change in a familiar pattern or behaviour and doesn't just refer to physical death. Loss is considered either physical or symbolic. Physical loss would of course include the death of another, but could also include the death of a pet or animal, experiencing a miscarriage, loss of hearing or sight, an amputation, or suffering from a debilitating illness that limits your physical ability. Physical losses can also be more material, such as losing a home due to a natural disaster. Symbolic loss, on the other hand, is seen as less tangible and could include any of the following: loss of a job, getting a divorce, retirement, placement in foster care, being abandoned by a friend or family member, losing a cherished dream, having a child leave home (empty nest syndrome) or loss of freedom after a long trip, a sabbatical or from being in 'lockdown' due to the coronavirus. Both types of loss can impact us physically, mentally, emotionally, behaviourally and socially, and both types of loss can also cause grief. You may have recently experienced a bereavement or other form of loss and be consciously aware that you are experiencing grief, the very reason you were drawn to buy this book. However, like myself, you may not realise that what you are experiencing right now is grief and may just feel stuck, unable to shift yourself out of a particular mental and emotional state. Whichever it is, conducting a Life Review will help you to consciously see your current levels of loss and begin to understand if you harbour any unprocessed loss and therefore unresolved grief within.

What is a Life Review?

A 'Life Review' is a very simple, insightful and rather logical right-brain exercise that requires a pen and paper. As the name suggests, it requires looking back over your life and noting any significant events and taking the time to honour your very unique path. I found the exercise fascinating and relatively quick to perform. Transforming the emotions connected to the events was a much longer process, which we will cover in the next chapter. The Life Review is simply like conducting your own version of *This is Your Life*—which, for those of you that are not old enough to remember, was a British biographical documentary TV show that ended over twenty years ago (I'm showing my age now). It involved a special celebrity guest being gifted with a big red book that detailed a timeline of events from their life. In chronological order, the presenter would take the guest on a journey through their life with the assistance of the timeline in the red book. It was filled with replaying memories, videos, photographs, news snippets, reporting on any special or memorable (good and bad) occasions or events that person had experienced. Sadly, conducting your own Life Review isn't quite as fancy, as you don't get given the big red book—you have to create it yourself. In fact, you don't even need a book—you just need a pen and paper, or if you prefer, remember you can download a free copy of the 'Mastering My Crown; Self Discovery Journal' and use that instead. Personally, I used two pages in a journal I was already using to track my weird anxiety and PTSD symptoms.

First, let's look at what type of events you might like to include in your own Life Review. Remember, the key point here is to look for change and periods of transition! Loss can come from the end of a familiar pattern or behaviour, so you are looking for any of the following:

* Changes in home/residence/country
* Changes in schools (Primary to Secondary, Sixth Form to University)
* Changes in job (role, location, promotion, retirement)
* Changes in boss or employer (not necessary a new role or job)
* Changes in work environment (relocating to a different site but with the same role or job)
* Changes in work staff (new team members coming or going)
* Changes in friends
* Changes in relationship status (endings and beginnings in relationships)
* Birth (family and friends)
* Death (family, friends, pets, famous idols such as musicians or actors)
* Marriage/Divorce
* Children (birth, adoption, miscarriage)
* Change in identity (name, gender or sex)
* Surgery or illness
* Trauma (physical, mental or emotional abuse, accidents)
* War (as civilian or military)
* Periods of stress (which would probably be caused by something on this list)

You may have experienced some other form of change and thus loss that isn't included in my list, but that's ok. Remember this is *your* Life Review.

How to Conduct a Life Review
So now you have an idea of what to include in your Life Review, you now need to source your pen and paper or Mastering My Crown; Self Discovery Journal. There are several methods to create your own Life Review and there is no right or wrong way, but the most important thing is not to miss or forget anything. I started at present day then chronologically worked backward, making a list down the page of any major events, emotionally moving experiences or changes I had experienced. My journal page looked a lot like this...

Panic Attacks & PTSD	2016
Dark Night of the Soul	2016
Nanny Cath Died	2016
Physical Pain and Sciatica	2015
2nd Spiritual Awakening	2015
Got Married	2015
Father Diagnosed with Prostate Cancer	2015
Adrian Died (A Friend's Husband)	2015
Hossein Moved In with Me	2015
Met Hossein	2014
Cervical Screening Abnormal Cells	2014
Ex-boyfriend Break Up	2014
Mum Diagnosed with Pulmonary Lung Fibrosis	2013
Met Lone-Wolf	2010
Ex-boyfriend Break-Up	2010
Michael Jackson Died	2009
Ex-boyfriend on Deployment to Afghanistan	2009

I continued this all the way to my birth, or more specifically to my first memory as a child. You don't have to include the year, but I did because I follow astrology and wanted to go back and check out what transits I was experiencing during these periods. You might find it easier to start by noting down any physical losses such as the death of family, friends or icons, miscarriages or debilitating changes to your physical health. Most people are aware of the year they experience such events. Then you could fill in the gaps with symbolic losses and any life changes. You might find that you think you have finished and then suddenly remember some life change you experienced and have to slot it in. You could even type the list using a computer as it's easier to edit and move things around. I was able to get all of mine onto two or three pages, but if you are older or have experienced more changes and loss throughout your life, your list will be longer.

In summary, here is a reminder of how to conduct a Life Review;

Equipment:
* Pen and Paper (I suggest using the Mastering My Crown: Self Discovery Journal).

 Instructions:
* List in chronological order any major losses (physical and symbolic), emotionally moving experiences and life changes.

 Top Tips:
* Allocate some time and space to conduct your Life Review.
* Remember, it's for your eyes only so it doesn't have to be neat and tidy.
* You may like to access old photo albums or personal documents to help you remember chronology.
* If you are already thinking your list will be too big, too time consuming or too overwhelming, just start small. Note down just two or three major losses and a few symbolic losses.

How to Use the Life Review

Once I had formulated my Life Review, I used a highlighter to mark any physical loss from bereavement, and immediately I saw a pattern. My first episode of panic attacks in my twenties started about two to three months after the passing of my Nanny Boobie (my mum's mum) and my more recent episode of panic attacks started two to three months after the passing of my Nanny Cath (my dad's mum). That's the first time I saw so clearly that death was my trigger. So, in the same way I did, perhaps use one colour marker to highlight any loss through physical death and another colour marker to highlight any symbolic loss. You might not have such startling insight right away like I did, but look for any themes, any periods of stress, illnesses that repeat or reoccur. Perhaps you can see a decline in your physical or mental health some months after a particularly emotionally moving experience.

Instead of seeing all the events of your life as seemingly unrelated moments in time, you can start to see your whole life as one interconnected web that has got you to where you are today. Now, armed with the knowledge that all change can bring a sense of loss and loss can cause grief, just look at the potential amount of unprocessed loss and repressed grief you may harbour within. So that is where we are going next... to explore grief, what it is, how it can manifest and— with the use of our Life Review—how to transform it.

CHAPTER 9

Understanding Your Grief

What is Grief?

Grief is the natural response following the loss of something or someone meaningful, either physical or symbolic, and is also the name given to the process of learning to cope with the loss experienced. Whereas mourning is the more outward expression of loss, grief includes the internal emotional response we feel on a very personal level. We could say that loss is the event or cause and grief is the outcome or effect. Although everyone will experience loss at some point in their lives, how you react to that loss and experience grief is unique to you, just like your fingerprint. In the case of physical loss, many factors can affect how grief can manifest, such as the circumstances surrounding a person's death and the relationship and attachment to that person. But remember, physical loss could also include a pet, so how long your pet had been part of your family and your relationship and bond with your pet will also play a part in that circumstance. In terms of physical and symbolic loss, our faith, religious or cultural beliefs, financial stability, mental health history, personality and a person's coping mechanism all contribute to how we experience grief. Remember back to the fear and stress response: Everyone has their own distinctive pressure gauge which will play a huge part in how you process grief.

Symptoms of Grief

Although grieving is a completely natural process that aids in our healing—the body's way of working through a mix of emotions—that doesn't make it any easier. Grief can be excruciating, especially in the acute initial stages, when it presents itself in many ways, especially emotionally. We may feel despair, anguish, sadness, sorrow, anger, rage, frustration, yearning, longing, fear, anxiety, emptiness, loneliness, helplessness, numbness, relief and confusion, etc. But it doesn't just affect our emotional state; grief can also impact our physical, mental, behavioural, social and spiritual selves too. We may experience insomnia, fatigue, confusion and disorganisation, preoccupied thoughts of the person who has passed, hallucinations, withdrawal, avoidance, loss of appetite or weight gain, a loss of faith, physical weakness, reduced immunity and even physical aches and pains. In some cases, we may even feel a sense of relief and solace when a family member or loved one dies, because they don't have to suffer any longer. This can bring up other emotions such as guilt and shame. Other times we may feel remorse or regret from words left unsaid; some people may even feel elation at the death of another, particularly if the relationship was abusive. We may also suffer from mental health issues such as panic attacks and depression, whether newly diagnosed or re-emerging from a previous mental illness diagnosis. Although during my grieving process I felt sad, hopeless and empty, I thankfully never felt suicidal. All I wanted to do was withdraw from the world and hibernate, I suppose to have a safe space where I could process all of my experiences. It's like my emotional world had flat-lined. I couldn't feel happiness or joy any longer, which is actually called anhedonia and can be a symptom of depression. Thanks to my spiritual team, by the time my PTSD subsided, I was already working on processing my grief, so I knew on some deeper level that how I was feeling was a natural process of emotional release. That's not to say I didn't have a chemical imbalance in my brain—I will never know whether I did—but I knew what the root cause was, so I wasn't worried about seeming depressed.

However, discerning between depression and grief can be confusing because they can overlap and create very similar symptoms such as sadness, a constant feeling of emptiness, insomnia and a lack of interest in life. All such symptoms are normal grief reactions, but the main difference tends to be the duration of the experience. Depression tends to be more constant and persistent, whereas grief tends to decrease over time and be experienced in cycles or waves relating to the deceased. Although there is no set timeframe for processing grief because it is highly personal, what's known as normal grief usually decreases in intensity after twelve months, once all the major anniversaries and holidays have been experienced by the bereaved. Normal grief is not considered a mental illness whereas depression is, so you can begin to see how confusion may arise. Personally, I believe that in many instances grief is mistaken for mild depression, especially grief caused by a symbolic loss where no bereavement occurs in the present time. As a result many people are medicated, which keeps them stuck in illness rather than taking responsibility for their emotional and mental state. If you are unsure whether you are experiencing grief or depression, please seek medical professional advice. Along with your current symptoms, your previous medical history and importantly your levels of loss, your doctor should be able to effectively diagnose and offer the correct course of treatment.

Duration of Grief
Since grief is unique to each person, the length of time spent grieving can be anywhere from weeks to months to years. There is no distinct timeframe and no predictable schedule. Some people unknowingly never fully grieve and so end up repressing their emotions, while others are consciously aware that they need to, but suppress and hold their emotions in. Grief tends to arise in cycles where you may have periods of reprieve followed by periods of emotional pain again. Initially, you may have more bad days than good, a sense of one step forward and two steps back, however as you work through your grief, you start to experience more of the good days. You may even start believing that you have processed all

of your grief, until *bam!*—out of nowhere you get knocked for six and you end up back feeling sad and empty again, sometimes feeling even worse than you did initially. I used to question whether it really was worse or whether it was just an illusion because I hadn't felt the awful feeling for so long. Sadly, we have been conditioned as humans to think in linear terms, but processing grief doesn't really have a definitive endpoint. As with all healing, it is a process with ebbs and flows, ups and downs, a continual spiral of contraction and expansion, light and darkness. I'm not sure we ever fully stop grieving, but there is a definite perception shift. We stop seeing the down days as bad and the up days as good, and we just learn to accept them as feelings that come and go. Learning to live with more love, appreciation and gratitude.

After some time I began to see a pattern in how my grief would manifest. I would experience chest and upper-back pain, pain that felt so physical I thought I kept injuring myself. But as soon as I purged my next bout of grief and released a load of emotions, the pain would vanish literally overnight. I would falsely believe that I had healed my grief until a few weeks later that tweaking in my upper-back muscles would arise, soon followed by the full-blown pain that would radiate from my shoulder blade then deep into the left side of my chest. As most people would, I began to fear something more severe was wrong, but I was told over and over again by my guides, 'It's healing from the past,' so I knew not to worry. I chose not to take painkillers too, because for me that would have felt like silencing my body's voice. Obviously I don't suggest anyone stops taking their prescribed pain medications; I just wanted to share this story so you can begin to understand that your physical body pains can be a reflection of unhealed emotional wounds and trauma.

Types of Grief
Whatever your experience of grief may be, try not to compare yourself to others, because there is no right or wrong way to

process it. You may hear things such as 'They were stricken or consumed with grief,' or hear people tell of being more upset and emotional with a pet dying than a parent. This is because grief is so diverse, and there are actually several types that you can encounter. Understanding which one you are experiencing at a specific point in your grieving process can help to shed further light on your healing and how best to process your emotions.

Normal Grief, as it's called, is a bit of a misnomer if you ask me, because as you now understand there really is no normal or standard experience of grief. I guess it's implying that when experienced, you will follow a broad range of symptoms that do lessen in intensity over time.

Anticipatory Grief is when we can begin to experience symptoms of normal grief before our loss happens. Family of terminally ill loved ones often begin emotionally detaching in preparation for a loved one's passing and can display feelings of guilt and/or controlling behaviours, almost to try and prevent the inevitable somehow. However, just because you began grieving before any physical loss occurs, doesn't mean you won't experience grief after a loved one's death. The dying person may also experience anticipatory grief.

Complicated Grief can arise in many ways when there is no resolution from the normal grieving process and as a result, grief becomes chronic and prolonged. A person becomes stuck in their emotional state, constantly reliving the loss and having ruminating thoughts about the person who has passed. Time does not seem to ease their pain and suffering. Although usually lasting more than twelve months, as I have previously mentioned, the timeframe for complicated grief can vary widely; therefore, the most important factor to consider is whether your normal daily functioning has been impaired. Substance abuse issues, co-dependency, unresolved trauma, adjustment disorders and other mental illnesses can all increase the likelihood of experiencing complicated grief.

In some cases complicated grief may warrant mental health intervention and medication, so again, if you are unsure please talk it through with your medical practitioner. Since the normal grieving process has become hindered in some way, the following types of grief can be experienced:

Absent Grief is where a person has an impaired response and shows no or few signs of distress from their grief. Just because someone isn't mourning, however, doesn't necessarily mean that they are not grieving. Remember, grief is the internal psychological reaction to loss. Shock, disbelief, denial and avoidance can all contribute to absent grief.

Abbreviated Grief can display as a somewhat short-lived period of processing where an individual can seem fine and to swiftly move on, like they have not actually taken the time to grieve. This can be due to experiencing anticipatory grief beforehand, or when something or someone immediately fills the void of a loss.

Delayed Grief manifests itself long after the loss has occurred. It could be triggered by something small or inconsequential, and those experiencing it may not be aware that their current emotional and mental state is due to unprocessed loss and repressed grief.

Distorted Grief is when there is an extreme reaction to loss, often accompanied with behavioural changes. Anger, resentment, rage and hostility towards oneself and others can occur. Tragic and unexpected loss often triggers such grief.

Disenfranchised Grief can occur when a loss is not acknowledged by those around the bereaved or is seen as unimportant. There is a minimising of the loss, which can create a sense of alienation and isolation. An example of disenfranchised grief is when a loved one suffers from Alzheimer's or dementia, so they are physically present but absent in other ways. Disenfranchised grief often occurs when a pet dies.

Exaggerated Grief can manifest as a more intense experience of normal grief that can be seen in a person's actions, words and mental health. They may exhibit self-destructive behaviours such as substance misuse and experience nightmares, abnormal fears, suicidal thoughts and the triggering of underlying psychiatric disorders.

Inhibited Grief can hide behind physical complaints such as upset stomachs, migraines and fatigue instead of the typical grief reactions. Grief can become inhibited when a person feels it inappropriate to express their grief, can't, or doesn't know how to due to their upbringing or personality.

Masked Grief can manifest as physical symptoms such as unusual behaviours or other negative habits not typical of a grieving person that impair day-to-day functioning. Masked grief and emotional suppression of feelings and emotions can be conscious or unconscious.

Secondary Grief is felt after the grief of the initial physical loss. A bereaved person may grieve the physical absence of a loved one and then also go on to grieve other aspects of their relationship, such as other roles that person took on in their life.

Cumulative Grief occurs when many losses are experienced within a short period, so you don't have the time to process each individual loss. When we experience many changes in our lives simultaneously, although we may think we are stressed due to physical symptoms, the cause may actually be emotional in nature due to loss and grief. Remember that repetitive activation of the fear/stress response (allostatic overload) has a detrimental effect on the physical body, eventually leading to a whole host of medical problems, and as a result, we end up trying to fix the body and not the emotions.

Traumatic Grief can arise when we experience a sudden and unexpected loss, such as from an accident, suicide, crime or terror attack. The contagious nature of the virus COVID-19 in most cases means that family members can't visit or be present as their loved one passes over, so their chance to say goodbye is taken from them. Such factors may add to the complexity of the normal grieving process and develop into more complicated grief.

Collective Grief is that which a group of people may experience when someone important in a community or country dies. Natural disasters, terror attacks and unexpected public and celebrity deaths can all cause collective grief. The tragic death of Princess Diana saw an outpouring of collective grief and mourning across the world, not just in the UK. Another example could include the more local Aberfan Disaster of 1966, a mining landslide which sadly killed a generation of Welsh school children.

Due to the worldwide spread of coronavirus, collective grief is not just being felt within communities and countries, but globally. At the time of writing, coronavirus has killed 127,260 people in the UK and over three million worldwide ($_{14}$), and I acknowledge all those lightworkers, healers, starseeds, Earth stewards, empaths, sensitives, etc. who are persistently transforming the continuing levels of collective fear and grief. Transmuting such heavy energy that surrounds the Earth and permeates the collective unconscious during this time is no small feat. You do this in service to humanity, and you understand it is the reason you came... but I see you, I feel you, and I honour each and every single one of you. After all, it is a choice, but you have stepped up to your purpose with commitment and dedication even when you have no acknowledgment for all of your work. To all those in prayer who offer continual love and compassion to others even in your differences, I bow to you too. Lastly, to you reading this book, I honour your courage and bravery, your willingness to step forward and transform your own personal grief. Please know that in healing your own grief, you are also helping to heal the collective. We are not separate.

Coping with Grief

Since grief can be expressed in many ways and affects every part of life, learning to cope with grief is essential. Firstly, understanding that grief is a very natural emotional response to loss and that the process can look very different for everyone is the first small but major step. Learning not to compare yourself to how others grieve and allowing yourself the time and space to let it unfold at a pace that is right for you is key. In today's Western culture, after the funeral and wake have taken place, after all the condolences, flowers, cards and other kind gestures, life goes back to normal for most. The immediate family, however, are left to begin paving a new life, one which now has a gaping hole in it. Although you might have caring friends and extended family, do seek out others who are experiencing or have experienced what is now your reality. Talk to them, share your feelings and thoughts and tell them of your love, your grief and your pain. Quite often, the bereaved feel like a burden and feel it inappropriate to keep mentioning their loved one who has passed. This can lead to isolation, further separation and loneliness, so having a support network around you is very important. You may even find yourself getting frustrated with some friends who seem to lack the ability to empathise and say the right thing. It is important at this point to remember that not everyone has experienced grief like yours; grief is highly individual. Also, many people shy away from it due to their own unprocessed loss and inability to work comfortably in the emotional realm. Open communication is important, and expressing how you feel helps to allow the emotions grief brings to the surface, ultimately transforming them. If you don't have a suitable friend to share your feelings with, perhaps try joining a like-minded group. These are now more likely to be conducted online due to social distancing measures, but there are so many forums and people coming together in bubbles of support. Appendix A lists some support helplines and resources that you may like to access, and remember, I have set up a free Facebook Support Group, Mastering Your Crown, for people working through this book.

Also, try to remain active. I don't mean go out and run a marathon—although some people do and raise funds for charities that hold special meaning—I just mean keep mobile. As you now understand, movement is so important not only to keep the physical body healthy but to also allow energy and emotions to keep flowing. Gentle walking or even some simple mobilising and stretching in the comfort of your own home will be beneficial to help in the grieving process.

Lastly, don't shame yourself for feeling a mix of emotions. This goes for people grieving and those with other mental health conditions. Although emotions can be complex and challenging, they are a part of being human, so don't worry if your emotions take you on a rollercoaster ride. Learning to let go and performing the 8 Step Sequence can help bring you back to balance, physically and emotionally.

The Stages of Grief
When my spiritual team kept telling me to explore grief, the first thing I came across was the traditional 'Five Stages of Grief' model devised by psychiatrist Elisabeth Kübler-Ross in 1969. The proposed five stages are:

* Denial – Where feelings of disbelief, confusion, numbness are felt
* Anger – Where feelings of frustration, anxiety, blame, projection are experienced
* Bargaining – Where you may struggle to find meaning in life, where you reach out, search or feel overwhelmed and lost
* Depression – Where emotional pain is felt as helplessness, sorrow and sadness and where detachment can occur
* Acceptance – Where you begin to feel hope and experience a rebirth

When I initially saw this model, it didn't really fit with how I was feeling and my experiences. Personally, my grief certainly didn't follow these stages chronologically and I didn't experience all the stages. Denial implies that we are resistant to the reality of what has happened, and—like a defence mechanism—can actually help to protect us against any shock. But I knew I wasn't in denial. Almost six months had passed since my Nan's passing, so I was aware that she was gone. I didn't feel angry either, and certainly hadn't pleaded with the universe to bring her back. I guess because of her old age, I had minimised her death in some respects, telling myself that she had lived a long and full life and had not had to suffer in the end.

Then there is the depression stage, and as I have previously explained, I didn't ever considered myself to be depressed. The only stage that made me stop and pause was the last stage... acceptance. Although I had logically accepted my Nan had died, I realised I was not accepting of death itself. The death of anything or anyone. So I was stuck.

Grief in Summary

Grief is a natural response to loss that can impact us emotionally, mentally, physically, behaviourally and socially. Grief is experienced differently by everyone, and a number of factors will play a part in the type of grief that manifests for you. Grief is not a mental illness, although it can trigger and cause mental health issues or develop into complicated grief disorder or complicated bereavement disorder. Your experience may or may not fit with the traditional five stages of grief, and it is definitely more complex when you start to look at symbolic loss. Until now, we have been mainly focused on grief following bereavement, but don't forget that grief is actually the natural response to any loss. However, mental and emotional states caused by symbolic loss are rarely recognised as grief. Technically, even the 'holiday blues' is a form of grief, since we are reacting emotionally to the end of a particular experience and behaviour, but it is a misconception to believe that grief is only caused by a loss that is not of your conscious doing. Grief, surprisingly, can also be caused by positive choices and changes you willingly make, such as taking a promotion, getting married, having a child, moving house, town or emigrating.

Using an analogy of a container of water, for each loss encountered, physical or symbolic, water is added to the container. Some people will quickly process the emotions connected to their loss and so their water level will fall almost immediately after being added. However, if water is continually added and never emptied, sooner or later it will reach the max line. At this point, you may notice yourself struggling to manage your mental and emotional health. You may even adopt some coping behaviours or try your best to remain in control.

Remember everyone's level of loss is different, so our water levels rise at different rates. For some, it can take years for the water to reach the max line, and for grief to fully manifest. Many people even think they have processed their losses or are unaware that they need to, until *whoosh*—all of a sudden the container is overflowing and a tidal wave of overwhelming emotions come rushing out in a sometimes uncontrollable and seemingly over-reactive manner.

Grief in 2020 and Beyond
For many people, 2020 has added a lot of water to their perhaps already full container. Perhaps you lost a parent as a child, but it was the loss of your current job that was just enough to make your container spill over. You may even feel confused as to why you are so emotional over losing a job you didn't like anyway, when really it was just the straw that broke the camel's back. Maybe you have been working from home due to the coronavirus, and loneliness has triggered some unresolved grief from a romantic relationship that ended some time ago. Maybe being told to wear a mask has triggered your memory of being overpowered and controlled by an abuser. Maybe having to abide by new rules and having your freedoms taken away by authorities has triggered deep ancestral wounding and multigenerational trauma held within your cells. Thanks to developments in epigenetics (the study of heritable changes in gene expression), increasing studies show what healers and shamans of ancient traditions have

always known: that memory gets passed down within our cells and DNA from one generation to next. Holocaust survivors, African Americans who experienced slavery, the descendants of the countless indigenous tribes, the Jewish community, women who were intuitive and psychic... all condemned and judged for their way of being. Like myself, you could have past life trauma that is playing out in your life now.

Whatever loss has caused your grief and whatever your symptoms, you can transform it. It wasn't something that I did overnight but a process that took time and patience, where I learned to adopt much self-compassion and self-acceptance. Now, you too can learn how to free yourself from your pain and suffering by learning how to transform your grief through 'Letting Go'.

CHAPTER 10

Understanding Letting Go

My 'Letting Go' Journey

I had been processing my grief through 'Letting Go' long before I mentally understood loss and grief. When I met my spirit guide Lone-Wolf in 2010, this opened up a portal into another world, another life, and with it came all the feelings and emotions from that life too. Experiencing his presence and feeling the most powerful and unconditional love from him also meant I was reminded what it was like to be without him. He passed when I was a young girl in my past life and I never fully grieved his death, so I was called to do it in this life. Thankfully, I have a wonderful father now too, but in finding myself with two loving fathers I experienced such a mix of emotions. They ranged from longing to utter gratitude, to then feelings of guilt because on some level it felt like I was betraying my father in this life. My husband was also a part of the same past life, so meeting him in my current life opened up a deep wound of separation. Although we were now physically brought together, my soul only knew life without him, and so this brought up many deep fears and painful wounding. It took me many years of self-healing to work through all the past cycles of longing, and had you asked me back then what I was feeling, I would have said overwhelming love and not loss. So much love I didn't know what to do with it all, and it wasn't until after my Dark Night of the Soul and PTSD that I realised I was grieving. By which time I was asked to explore my loss from this lifetime too, which needed a completely different approach, but thanks to the help of Angel Ezekiel in conducting my Life Review, I knew exactly where to start.

Since I saw an immediate connection between physical death and my panic attacks, I felt called to start my 'Letting Go' process here first. In reverse chronological order, with the most recent bereavement first, I began to process any emotions I held connected to each loss. I started with a rather logical and right-brained exercise of writing my Nan a letter. I made sure I choose a time I wasn't going to be disturbed and then, with pen and paper, began 'Dear Nan...', firstly telling her how I was feeling. I didn't hold back either. I told her how her death had made me question my life and myself. I told her how it opened up a deep fear within me and how I felt scared, even sorry that I hadn't fully understood what was happening when her energy came to me as she passed over.

Being a psychic medium, you may wonder why I didn't just have a conversation with her in spirit. Well, that's because during my Dark Night of the Soul, my energy contracted so much from fear that I was unable to communicate with my guides or spirit for this period. Plus, this was part of my learning, to feel somewhat abandoned in order to hear only my own shadow energy talking.

Anyway, in the letter I asked her to forgive me if I'd done anything wrong or if I could have helped her more in some way. I thanked my Nan for all she had done for me when I was younger... the long walks she used to take my brother and me on, for her 'goodie cupboard' full of jelly moulds and refrigerated pink mouse. I told her that I loved her and needed to let all my painful emotions go but that by doing so I wasn't forgetting her, then I said goodbye. I cried as I wrote the letter and re-read it several times for a few days after; sometimes I felt emotional and other days I felt nothing. You may remember from my earlier writing that this only brought short-term relief, and I found my dark, flat and sad mood returned again soon after, and I became stuck. Thankfully, that's when Angel Ezekiel imparted his wisdom and helpful guidance, opening up my awareness of loss and grief, which led to a realisation that I would need to apply the same process to all of my current life's losses. So once I had written my letters to each and every person I had physically lost through death, I moved on to symbolic losses, starting with romantic relationships. Each letter I wrote, although following the same format, was very different, a reflection of the different kind of relationship and connection I'd had with each of those I had lost. The letters to previous romantic partners were very different from those I had written for family because the feelings I shared weren't always what we would consider as 'positive'. In some instances I included how I felt angry, rageful, emotionally abused, betrayed, taken for granted, unheard... the list goes on. However, when I delved deeper, underneath it all I simply found hurt, vulnerability, abandonment, loss and grief.

Everyone has a core wound, and in most cases it involves some form of abandonment at the most fundamental level. This abandonment is what creates separation and loss, both of which cause grief, the complex emotion that is often disguised as anger, pain, resentment, bitterness, rage, frustration, hurt etc. Interestingly, for the first time in maybe twenty years, I saw my first ever boyfriend the very day after writing my 'Letting Go' letter to him. Many would say that it was a coincidence, but I knew it was a synchronicity and a little wink from the universe to confirm I was now heading in the right direction.

Just to clarify, you don't actually have to give the letter to the person you have written to, and they don't have to physically read it for it to take effect. Energy is not bound by space and time. In fact, in some cases giving your written letter to another could create added complications, conflict and more energetic attachments.

Next, I wrote letters to those who were physically still present in my life and would continue to be even after the 'Letting Go' process. This included writing letters to my mum, my dad, my husband and the most difficult of all... a letter to myself. Please don't think that performing such 'Letting Go' practices means that you will physically separate from the person in question or that they will be removed from your life. It doesn't work that way. Anyone who needs to be in your life for you to live out your purpose and learn your lessons will remain— that goes for anyone you choose to keep in your life as well. It just frees up space to allow the relationship to evolve and grow from a healthier place. Although my mum is still alive, I wrote a letter to her regarding her health condition... who she was before it compared to who she is now. I wrote a letter to my husband, the man I married compared to the man he has become. You see, we have to allow people to be exactly who they are and not limit and confine people to our own perceptions and expectations. Every person has the right and free will to change and evolve or, in some cases, not. You may not like the change or lack of, and it may not be in line with what you want or desire, but they are allowed to be exactly who they want to be. That is the true nature of the spiritual path... to open your heart to unconditional love, which means loving with no conditions! It's by no means an easy path and involves making tough choices, such as whether to continue giving your time, dedication, energy and love to another or not.

Lastly, I came to work through my personal symbolic losses, such as leaving my job, my marriage and my own mental health problems, which actually at their root were about losing myself. The loss of my ego structures, my name and my purpose, which all reflected the changing person within. Interestingly, to others looking from the outside, I probably hadn't seemed to have changed at all. I hadn't drastically changed my hair or moved countries, but my inner world had been transformed beyond recognition. When I finally said goodbye to Emma Bradshaw, it allowed Emma Gholamhossein the room to birth.

What is 'Letting Go'?

Letting go is a simple action. If you are holding a ball in your hand and are instructed to let it go, your thought and will join together and you make a choice to loosen your grip. The muscles respond and the ball then drops to the floor. We say you have let go. It's a conscious choice of action that happens in an instant. Now, think about the same scenario, only this time the ball is the last thing that you and your father played with before he died suddenly. You may find it harder to drop the ball because those memories of him flood back, or maybe you fear that a dog might swoop in and run away with it, preventing you from picking it back up. Suddenly, the simple act of letting go becomes much more complex, fraught with worries, anxieties, emotions and fears.

In the first scenario, we knew exactly what would happen: we would let go and the ball would fall to the floor, where it would remain. However, we didn't see the possibility of a dog running in to snatch it because we held no fear regarding being able to pick it back up. The ball held no significance or meaning to us, so we had no emotional attachment to it. When we hold emotional attachments to people, places and objects, etc., the act of letting go becomes more difficult. In truth, instead of simply dropping the ball, we have to face all the fears that prevent us from doing so before the simple act of letting go can occur, and this requires conscious choice and action.

What are Emotions?

Please take a moment and consider: what are emotions to you? What are your perceptions and views regarding emotions? Do you think they should be expressed whenever they are felt? Is there a time and a place for expressing emotions? Which emotion do you feel and express the most? Do you feel that emotions take over and prevent you from being able to express yourself clearly? Would you try and prevent yourself from crying in front of another? Can you even cry at all? Are you uncomfortable if someone gets upset in your presence? If so, how do you respond? Do you find yourself saying, 'stop crying'? Are you naturally emotional, or would you consider yourself emotionally closed off? Are you comfortable to show anger, frustration or confidence but less comfortable showing confusion, uncertainty and vulnerability? Would you like to be able to express your emotions more? Where do these beliefs and habits originate? Are they really yours or habits you have been taught?

Try not to simply just read over these questions, giving them a fleeting thought only. Actually sit with them, contemplate them, even try to answer them on paper.

Self-development work isn't always comfortable. It's like peeling layers of an onion, and that can sting and bring tears to the eyes! Sadly, modern society—especially the very British 'Keep Calm and Carry On' motto—has taught us to believe that we shouldn't show our emotions and vulnerabilities and that doing so somehow makes us weak. Males are particularly hard hit by such damaging stereotypical beliefs. Even New Age spiritualism has incorrectly taught us to believe that we should only think positive thoughts and that negative 'low vibe' or 'low frequency' thoughts and emotions should be avoided. 'Love and light' is a wonderful ethos to live by, but only when one is equally willing to use that light to shine into their own darkness. Even the 'Law of Attraction' has in many cases created further delusion, inadvertently promoting the bypassing of our very real emotional nature. To be human is to feel, and life is about experiencing all the pains and pleasures that it brings. When we can look past the polarised and dualistic notion that something must be good or bad and look at things from a perspective of soul growth, we learn to be more accepting of ourselves and of others. Non-attachment to good versus bad helps us to accept the very changing nature of our world and of our emotional nature.

There is much debate in the scientific community about how to define emotion, but most agree that emotions are chemical reactions in response to our interpretation of an internal or external event. If you remember back to the fear response, the brain perceives danger which creates physiological changes in the body with chemical neurotransmitters and hormones. Fear is just one distinct human emotion, but other well-known basic emotions are happiness, surprise, sadness, anger and disgust, all of which affect our feelings and mood. Recently, in 2017, scientists discovered as many as 27 distinct categories of emotion ($_{15}$), some of which include envy, boredom, horror, nostalgia, sexual desire and triumph. Some emotions such as bitterness are actually a complex layering of emotions including disappointment, disgust, anger and fear. So although we are specifically focused on processing grief, another complex multi-layer emotion, please don't be alarmed if you begin to experience other feelings rising. While emotions are simply unconscious and automatic reactions, our feelings around those emotions are much more subjective, driven by our thoughts and past experiences.

But whatever you resist persists, so learning to let go of your emotions and feelings and not holding on to them will liberate you from the pain that they can bring. In doing so, you will begin to reshape and remould your current experience, which over time helps transform your thoughts, beliefs and expectations too. You will begin to manifest a reality based on your heart's desire, not what your conditioned emotional response and behaviour creates. By healing your grief, you are improving your self-awareness and developing emotional intelligence, a wisdom that can't regress, because once your consciousness expands it can't go backwards. This means you are growing and evolving— and that, my friends, is the purpose of this life... to learn, to live and to be a better person than you were yesterday. But as is the nature of the universe, both positive and negative polarities exist. We expand, but we must also learn to contract. We rise up, but only through learning to go within. All is in balance then.

How to Write a 'Letting Go' Letter

In order to process your grief, you are required to first explore any held emotions and feelings about your loss. Writing a 'Letting Go' letter helps to access such feelings and requires the utmost self-honesty and bravery when facing whatever emotions and feelings arise, whether you perceive them as good or bad. Remember, feeling emotions is simply part of being human, and just like clouds in the sky, they should come and they should go. It's when they get stuck that complications can arise, so you want to keep them fluid so they can be processed in a non-destructive way. Knowing how to stabilise yourself if and when you feel emotionally overwhelmed is also key, and that's why performing the 8 Step Sequence alongside this process is essential to help keep yourself balanced and centred.

 Instructions:

1. **Source some paper and a pen**
   You could use your Mastering My Crown; Self Discovery Journal or your current diary if you wish.

2. **Create a safe and sacred space**
   Make sure you have enough time where you won't be disturbed. Choose a location to be alone. It might be in the comfort, privacy and security of a room in your own home, or you might choose the car or the beach. You might like to light a candle, burn some sage or incense and even play some gentle music. You might like to have a picture of your loved one or a special object that holds significant meaning. You might not want to do any of those things and just get on with the process. There is no right and wrong here, just your personal preference.

3. **Perform the 8 Step Sequence**
   If feeling apprehensive and nervous or emotionally overwhelmed at the thought of writing your 'Letting Go' letter, I suggest performing the 8 Step Sequence to help you calm and centre yourself before you commence.

4. **Choose a loss from your Life Review**

Although I started the 'Letting Go' process with loss from physical death before moving onto symbolic loss, please don't feel you have to begin this way. Trust in your own knowing and gut feeling here... that will know where to start. You may feel a real deep resistance and repulsion from one particular loss, and that is fine—perhaps you are not ready to go there. In that case start smaller, start with some less significant loss and build up your confidence with using this process. Learning to trust yourself is part of this process, and you won't always get it right, but that's ok because we learn from the choices we make.

5. **Write your 'Letting Go' letter**

You might be tempted to follow your own format when writing your 'Letting Go' letter. However, there are important reasons why they should be structured in the following manner which we discuss later:

* Like you would a traditional letter, start with 'Dear/To' followed by their name. Please be mindful that the name you chose will affect the 'Letting Go' process. You may use their nickname, their full name or other intimate terms of endearment that were special between you, but remember we all have ego structures where we acquire certain roles and adopt certain behaviours. Some people use different names for these ego structures and in different capacities such as at home or in work. So although you might be letting go of the grief and emotions you hold towards your ex-partner, for example, who you called by a nickname, that is just one aspect of their being. The same way we label someone Mum, Dad, brother or sister, etc., underneath those roles and labels, they are someone much bigger, they are a whole person. So I advise considering carefully which name you choose. Perhaps you will need to write two letters to different aspects of their being or include all their names on one letter.

* Now you are going to share every thought you want with the person in question. All the words left unspoken, all the things you avoided saying to keep the peace, all the love you still have for them which you are no longer able to express. Importantly, tell them how you feel about them.
* 'I miss you because...' or 'I'm angry with you because...'. Equally, it might be sad, relieved, bitter, resentful, shameful, misunderstood, heartbroken, unforgiving, shattered, in pain, in disbelief, in shock, happy, grateful, etc. You could start with... 'You made my life wonderful because...' or 'You hurt me because...'
* The content and theme of the letter will really be guided by your unique relationship with the person you have lost (whether through physical or symbolic loss).
* Once you feel you have poured your heart out and have said everything you want to say, know that you have already started to transform the emotions connected to your loss. However, some will need further assistance to go deeper.
* If at this point you are overly emotional from writing your 'Letting Go' letter, I advise taking a pause to allow the emotions and subsequent thoughts to percolate and settle. It may be at this point you begin to experience other emotions you were not expecting to feel. You see, once energy has shifted, a period of stabilisation is needed where you find your footing in your new awareness.
* Perform the 8 Step Sequence regularly to help foster stabilisation in your new awareness and reality.
* Once you feel you have had sufficient respite or if you feel stable emotionally and mentally after writing your 'Letting Go' letter, you are ready to proceed to the next stage of the 'Letting Go' process, whereby you become the alchemist.

CHAPTER 11

Becoming the Alchemist

Alchemy is a practice and philosophy originating from Ancient Egypt that believed certain chemical processes could transmute base metals into gold. Thankfully, you don't need any test tubes or a white coat to become the modern-day alchemist of your inner world. Remember, emotions, memories and beliefs are all stored deep within our nervous system, our immune system, our muscles and cells, so writing the 'Letting Go' letters help to access any unconsciously held emotions. When we express them, we share what was repressed (unconsciously held in) and suppressed (aware of but consciously held in). For some, simply writing the letter where they conceptualise their feelings and convert their stored emotions into words is enough to release them. However, others will need to go deeper to really connect to their words and innermost feelings and transform them.

Transforming Emotions
Emotions are simply energy in motion and that energy cannot be destroyed only transformed from one form to another. In order to transform emotions fully after accessing them through the 'Letting Go' letters, we must allow them to lift up and out of the subconscious, which means becoming aware and conscious of them. This means feeling them. This won't always be nice, but it is necessary. To heal we need to feel. You might find yourself facing deep fears and other emotional complexities that are standing in the way of you letting go. The way through this is to foster acceptance, forgiveness, repentance, gratitude, love and surrender.

Acceptance

Fundamentally, acceptance is recognising and consenting to something without attempting to change it. It means fully embracing the present, however that may look. When we are not ready to embrace acceptance, we may still fight against or avoid our current reality. Although acceptance is a state that we aim to reach, it also involves noticing oneself when in resistance and fighting mode. It doesn't mean that you stop feeling that mix of emotions; it just means that you become mindful of where you are. By noticing, you can then choose to adopt more healthy thoughts and behaviours from your new emotional awareness.

Repentance

Repentance simply means to be genuinely sorry for something that you have done, such as nasty words you said in anger or action you took out of spite. It could mean being sorry for causing physical, emotional, mental or spiritual suffering or harm to another. Now, like myself, you may be thinking, 'Well, I'm nice, I haven't got anything to be sorry for because I haven't hurt anyone.' However, sometimes we can hurt another unknowingly, without intent or purpose. So repentance is showing and feeling sincere regret and remorse for anything you may have done unintentionally that caused harm or distress for another. You may even feel yourself reject the idea of needing to repent, and if so, I say this... Although you may perceive yourself as 'proper and good' in this life, your soul may have intentionally hurt another in a past incarnation. I speak from experience here, so repentance is for all.

Forgiveness

Forgiveness is a conscious deliberate decision to release feelings of resentment, bitterness, guilt or vengeance towards yourself or another that may have caused you emotional hurt, pain and suffering either knowingly or unknowingly. To forgive does not mean to forget, nor does it mean condoning or excusing a person for any hurt they have caused. It just means you are no longer willing to carry around the negative emotions and baggage, and are moving from hostility and aggression to cooperation and conciliation. Although we think of forgiveness as an act, it is also a state that we can continually adopt, and by embracing a forgiving mindset, symbolic losses such as changes in the health of a loved one may be more easily processed. Practices that foster forgiveness for some may have negative connotations attached to them due to religious undertones, however science has now found growing evidence to support such practices in positively influencing mental health ($_{16}$).

Gratitude
Gratitude is a feeling of appreciation and thankfulness towards the world at large, someone or something specific. Gratitude, along with joy and love, is one of the highest vibrational states one can experience and connects you directly to what I call divine source and creation energy. When we like something or a gesture someone has made, it is easy to feel grateful, but when we have an experience that we don't like, it's more difficult to foster gratitude. Although many people see gratitude as a temporary emotional state, like mindfulness and forgiveness, it can also be adopted as a daily practice. Having a grateful and positive mindset is incredibly powerful. However, toxic positivity and gratitude can be harmful, especially as a means for avoiding uncomfortable emotions.

Love
Love means different things to different people, and there are many different types of love. The platonic love we feel for a friend or family member, the passionate love we feel for a romantic partner, etc. We say we love something when it gives us a feeling of happiness or joy, or when someone or something makes our lives easier, more meaningful and more complete. The Ancient Greeks had eight words that were used to express the different types of love one can experience. 'Eros' love is that of a passionate nature that we can experience with a romantic partner. 'Mania' is a type of love where you become obsessive and intoxicated with another. 'Philia' is an affectionate and platonic love

that includes a kind of mutual respect between two people. 'Storge' is a type of love that feels familiar, perhaps the one we experience with emotionally close family and friends. 'Ludus', or playful love, can be expressed as flirtation and with no depth of emotional attachment. 'Philautia', or self-love, is that which we consider beneficial for our own well-being rather than that of vanity and selfishness. 'Pragma', or enduring love, is considered practical and founded on duty, whereby a relationship matures over many years. Lastly, 'Agape', or selfless love, is considered the highest form of pure love that is universal and unconditional. The spiritual path leads to the ability and want to love in this way, whereby a person's growth and evolution is considered most important. It is also the love connected to the thymus gland, higher heart and crown chakras.

Surrender and Goodbye

In acceptance, we chose to let go and therefore have some control. It is an action for the ego because we consciously allow it with our logical mind and take action with our will. In surrender, there is a complete letting go of control. In life, there are just certain things that we simply cannot control, and for the most part, we certainly can't control when someone we love dies, so we have to surrender to that fact. Only when we fully accept the fundamental nature of our world and universe, which follows a changing pattern of contraction then expansion, of birth then decay, can we truly surrender. In surrender there is a yielding, a 'giving up' and 'giving way' to something bigger than our self, so we submit and stop trying. That's when letting go finally takes place, in an instant, like in the simple act of dropping a ball from your hand, but it's human nature to resist this. Surrender is not weakness, but a sign of strength. It takes the utmost bravery to let go of control. Only with faith, trust, knowing and acceptance of the impermanence of all life can we truly let go and say goodbye to what was and has been, because we come to realise that there is really no death, only ever transformation and rebirth. When we let go, we don't end there; we continue, and something new will be born from that ending.

Goodbye, however, doesn't mean 'out of sight out of mind'. It means that we allow ourselves to move on, to be free to live again without any heavy emotional burdens, restrictions and limitations. With every ending comes a new beginning, and that is fundamentally the highest expression of the feminine energy: letting go of the old so the new can be born. The highest expression of the masculine energy then is sustaining what happens in the middle. Two different jobs but of equal importance. For millennia, people have feared the power of the feminine energy, because fundamentally it involves the unknown—death—but when we lose our fear of surrender, just like Mother Earth herself, we begin to achieve stability through constant change and transformation.

Transforming Emotion Affirmations
As with all manifestation work, simply using the power of the mind or thinking you want something to happen isn't enough. For example, thinking 'I want to release this grief,' using the conscious mind won't transform and change that emotion. You need to become the alchemist and transform it yourself. Remember, energy cannot be destroyed, so when you let go of an emotion, it has to go somewhere. It is far better to convert and transform that energy in motion (e-motion) into another form that is more beneficial. So the negative emotions and feelings that manifest as grief really just need to be transformed into other more beneficial emotions, and the simplest method to do this is with the use of affirmations. That is a process of self-empowerment by stating something to be true, and here is what you need to do...

✏️ Instructions:

1. **Read your 'Letting Go' letter aloud**
   Reading and speaking your written text and words aloud holds more power. The mental realm of consciousness and thought is unseen and unknown to others (unless you are telepathic or can read energy, of course), so by speaking the words aloud you are physically manifesting energy in the form of sound.

2. **Now state the following aloud – 'I accept'**
   'With all that I am, I accept all that has been and all that is. I accept all I have written in this letter, and I accept everything exactly as things are now. For any ways in which I am not ready to accept, I forgive myself.'

3. **Now state the following aloud – 'I am sorry'**
   'With all that I am, I am sorry. I am sorry for any suffering and pain I may have caused you physically, emotionally, mentally or spiritually, either knowingly or unknowingly. For any ways in which I am not ready to be sorry, I forgive myself.'

4. **Now state the following aloud – 'I forgive'**
   'With all that I am, I forgive you. I consciously choose to forgive you for any physical, emotional, mental or spiritual pain you have knowingly and unknowingly caused me. For any ways in which I am not ready to forgive you, I forgive myself.'

5. **Now state aloud – 'I am grateful'**
   'With all that I am, I am grateful for you. I am grateful for all the lessons you taught me, even the ones I didn't want. For any ways in which I am not ready to be grateful, I forgive myself.'

6. **Now state aloud – 'I love you'**
   'With all that I am, I love you, I send love and I am love. For any ways in which I am not ready to give or accept love from myself or others, I forgive myself.'

7. **Now state aloud – 'goodbye'**
   'With all that I am, I fully let you go, (insert name). Goodbye.'
   Now visualise yourself simply letting go of the ball from in your hand.

8. **Perform the 8 Step Sequence to finish**
   This will help stabilise the mind, body, emotions and subtle energies.

You may do this once and instantly feel the transformation taking place. However, like myself, you may find that you need to repeat the affirmations several times to really connect to the words, allowing yourself to feel their meaning. Simply repeating the affirmations verbatim won't cut it; you need to believe what you are saying, so pay attention to how your body reacts when you state each of them. Notice where you feel resistance. You may find that you can easily transform your hurt into forgiveness, for example, but find accepting love more difficult. Remember this process will take time, and practising radical self-forgiveness as you move through it will help to release any blocks more quickly. Only recently, while performing a healing session for another, I received guidance for her that involved forgiveness, and as a consequence I came to discover an ancient Hawaiian healing technique known as Ho'oponopono (pronounced ho-ah-po-no-pono). It greatly resembles the process I intuitively undertook in the unravelling of my grief and transforming the emotions connected to it. I only mention it for your information, should you wish to research further. It simply reconfirms to me that the new age is simply the re-emerging of the old and that most concepts are not new, just recycled and experienced in different ways. Energy, after all, cannot be created nor destroyed, just transformed.

In summary, here is a reminder of how to transform your Grief;

Equipment:
* Pen and Paper (I suggest using the Mastering My Crown: Self Discovery Journal).

Instructions:
* Write a 'Letting Go' letter to all those who you have physically lost through death, explaining how you feel about them and your relationship.
* Write a 'Letting Go' letter to all those who you have lost through change (end of a relationship, friend moving away, etc.) explaining how you feel about them and your relationship.
* Write a letter to yourself explaining how you feel about yourself (the old you before experiencing a specific change or loss).

Format:
* Dear/To... (Add appropriate name/names)
* I feel... because...

Affirmations:
* Read your 'Letting Go' letter aloud then state the full transforming affirmations for:
* I accept
* I am sorry
* I forgive
* I am grateful
* I love you
* Goodbye

Top Tips:

* Don't rush the process of writing your 'Letting Go' letters. Write one at a time, conducting the transforming affirmations for each person before moving onto writing your next 'Letting Go' letter.
* This is not a tick-box exercise; you need to engage with the process and allow yourself to feel what you are writing.
* Although the process of writing a letter following a specific format is straightforward, your emotions are not logical so won't necessarily arise in a logical pattern.
* Remember your letters are for your eyes only, so they don't have to be neat and tidy.
* You do not have to give the physical letter to the person it is addressed to for the 'Letting Go', release and closure to take place. In fact, doing so could create more challenges, conflicts and problems.
* Don't force the process. Be gentle and allow it to unfold at the correct pace for you.
* The transforming emotion affirmations are very specific, which aids in the 'Letting Go' process. However, please don't be tempted to change them. Instead, please feel free to add to them.
* Although the second half of this book is specifically aimed at releasing and transforming the emotions connected to grief, the same process can be used for any relationships to aid in conflict resolution.
* It is extremely important to remember that this is a process and transforming your emotions will take time. Please do not berate yourself if you cannot fully accept, forgive, be sorry, be grateful and love initially. The most important thing here is practising radical self-forgiveness, because such compassion, surrender and allowing helps to dissolve the fears and blocks that stand in your way of 'Letting Go'.

IMPORTANT NOTE

* Once you have completed this whole process (written 'Letting Go' letters and stated the transforming emotion affirmations) for your grief, I highly suggest completing the process with letters for your parents (biological, adoptive and/or caregiver), regardless of whether you still see them, they are still alive or have ever been in your life. The most fundamental underlying wound in all humans is abandonment, and for many there can be unresolved emotions relating to the 'Father' and 'Mother' principle. Such wounding not only plays out in the lives of children but can manifest well into adulthood, affecting your current relationships.

Transmuting Energetic Attachments and Patterns

Although you may have transformed all the emotions connected to a certain person as they pertain to your current life, you may still hold a particular energetic imprint, pattern or attachment that keeps you stuck and unable to let go, transform and rise again, fully transmuted as a new version of yourself. We not only carry trauma that gets passed down from one generation to the next but also patterns, beliefs, behaviours and attitudes that continue in the bloodline until they are healed and released.

Over the last six years, I have been called to heal my own bloodline and multigenerational trauma. Firstly, from my dad's side of the family, who were more emotionally detached, and then my mum's side, who were emotionally sensitive and overwhelmed. Also, nearly every energy healing session I have performed on another included healing ancestral family wounds and patterns. Although the person lying on my treatment couch would be the one who came for healing, their parents, grandparents, great-grandparents even, would also show up for healing too. Sometimes these relatives and ancestors were in spirit, other times they were still very much alive, but part of their multidimensional energy—unknowingly, of course—was with us. I saw so many people who were stuck and experiencing problems with their health, an inability to conceive a child, relationship conflicts, an inability to let someone or an unhealthy habit go, etc., and really the problem wasn't theirs.

Don't get me wrong—we can't blame everything on our parents and bloodline. We always have free will and possibly karmic debt to repay, so energetic attachments and patterns stemming from actions we took in past lives. For example, any vows, promises, contracts, pledges or oaths that have been made in this life or previous lives that have not been fulfilled still hold energetically. That's why being honourable and clear with your word is important, because words carry vibration and power. They are the spells we cast on ourselves and others; the word 'spelling' actually means forming words with letters. Sometimes, I am called to cut etheric cords, which are energetic links between certain people, not dissimilar to a single piece of rope connecting them together. The etheric cords, however, come in different thicknesses and textures and can be connected to anywhere in the aura, chakra or even energetically inside a person. You see, when we are energetically connected to others via etheric cords, they can siphon off our own energy and almost imprint a certain pattern and programme, keeping us in a negative and repetitive loop or cycle. Patterns that replay over and over. Much like how a computer runs the same program every time you turn it on until you update it or install a new program. You may no longer have communication with the person in question—they could be in spirit, for example, so no longer physically in body—but energetically you may still be connected. So they may still have some hold over you in some way, even unconsciously and unknowingly.

Transmuting Energetic Attachment and Pattern Affirmations
Just like you were able to transform your emotions, you can also transmute any energetic attachments, patterns and programmes using affirmations.

✏️ Instructions

1. **Set aside some time and space to be alone**
   To honour your spirit and your unique soul journey, you might like to light a candle or play some empowering music, or you may prefer to visit your favourite place.

2. **Perform the 8 Step Sequence**
   This will help to bring balance to your body, mind, emotions and energy, and you will be better able to focus on the task at hand.

3. **State the following aloud:**
   * 'I, (insert full name), disconnect from and release any energy that is not my own.'
   * 'I, (insert full name), recall all of my energy back home to myself.'
   * 'I, (insert name), am a full sovereign being and relinquish and denounce any vows, oaths, promises or verbal declarations I have ever made across all time, space and dimensions that no longer serve my highest good.'
   * 'I, (insert name), am a full sovereign being, and I relinquish and command the end of any karmic ties, connections or contracts across all time, space and dimensions that no longer serve my highest good.'
   * 'Thank you, it is done.'

4. **Now, simply allow whatever unfolds and drop any expectations that you may have**
   Know that you have the power and authority to make any change you wish at any time. Your life is now your own and you are regaining your sovereignty.

PART 3:

Mastering Your Crown

CHAPTER 12

Additional Guidance

Although certainly not the main feature of the book, this chapter shares important but additional guidance and information to help you better manage your anxiety, fear, loss and grief.

Distraction Techniques

Distraction techniques can include watching a movie, phoning a friend, crosswords, puzzles, doodling, reading a book or counting objects in your immediate environment that are a certain colour or begin with a particular letter of the alphabet, etc. They help to occupy the conscious mind and redirect our attention away from any unpleasant symptoms, sensations or intrusive thoughts we may be experiencing. During my periods of dissociation and depersonalisation, I used to try and distract myself from the feeling of impending doom and weird sense of my body dissolving. At the time, I didn't fully understand these were symptoms of my fear response, so I would panic more, plus my mind was so burnt out I couldn't concentrate or focus on anything that required any real effort. Equally, my body was so hypervigilant and sensitised that I had to be very particular with what I watched on the TV (a distraction technique I had barely used before). Anything that was even remotely emotionally moving or thrilling was a no-go for me because it would cause me to have a panic attack. I couldn't even listen to music when I first had PTSD, because I found it too stimulating. Personally, although I did try such distraction techniques, the relief was only short-lived, because as soon as the distraction finished, I was still left with weird sensations that seemed to return with greater vengeance. You see, distracting yourself aimlessly without any real outcome only serves as a quick fix for managing symptoms of anxiety rather than a standalone solution to mental illness recovery. Over time, I began to realise that by distracting myself I was simply masking the issue, covering up the weird sensations instead of getting to the root cause of them. That's when I knew there had to be another way and I was guided to begin 'Sensing' my feet and patting down my body and found myself performing the Medulla Hold. I hadn't developed the full 8 Step Sequence at this point, but I suggest you use that as your distraction technique in itself.

 Top Tips
* Experiment with different types of distraction techniques.
* Try Googling funny clips/videos that make you laugh. This helps to reduce the body's fear/stress response and releases endorphins, the body's feel-good hormones.
* Use the 8 Step Sequence as your distraction technique.

Grounding and Earthing

I have seen the term 'grounding' used to incorrectly describe 'Sensing' for relief from anxiety and panic attacks and wanted to discuss this topic briefly. Bringing your attention to your immediate environment by noticing a fragrance you can smell, objects you can see, sounds you can hear and textures you can feel can all have a profoundly relaxing effect on the mind and body. This is because you are drawing all of your awareness to a focus point and your senses are bringing your attention back to your immediate environment. However, these techniques are more correctly termed 'Sensing', which forms Step 4 in the 8 Step Sequence. Remember, Sensing opens up our mind-body connection, both our exteroceptive systems such as hearing, smell, touch, sight and taste and our interoceptive systems—those we use to perceive our internal state, such as pain and heat. However, because Sensing helps to centre oneself, people often say they are 'grounded' in the present moment, which is an expression for how they are feeling following Sensing.

The more common term 'grounding', as known in the spiritual/New Age community, actually refers to an exercise whereby you image having tree roots that are attached to your feet that grow down into the Earth. This type of grounding exercise has many benefits. Firstly, it helps to focus the mind. Secondly, it opens up your sensing abilities, and thirdly, it helps the flow of your energy polarity from the head, through the body and legs to the feet, so positive to negative charge. 'Grounding' can be done in several ways, including through visualisation/imagery, attention/focus, and using mudras, which are specific hand positions that help direct energy flow. You can even practise breathing through your feet, which is a highly relaxing and powerful way to ground your energy. Spiritually, grounding also helps to connect with Mother Earth, sometimes known as Gaia, the primordial living goddess and mother of all life in Greek mythology.

Humanity as a whole has disconnected from the mother/ female principle in favour of the father/masculine, which can be seen through the ruling patriarchal societies, world powers and religions. Mother Earth, the planet and home of the human race, has been raped and pillaged of her resources, her waters and air polluted, her inhabitants (creatures, plants and animal species) killed. An overreliance on masculine energy has resulted in wars, power struggles and unsustainable choices that have caused much environmental damage. Connecting to the feminine principle helps to bring greater balance and order within, and thus to our outer world where the masculine energy has until now dominated.

I have also seen the term 'Earthing' used interchangeably with 'grounding', but there is a distinct difference. 'Earthing' means putting the body in direct and uninterrupted contact with the Earth. From a scientific perspective, the idea is that the Earth has a mild negative charge to it, and when we put our positively charged bodies in direct contact with it, Earth evens out this positive charge and returns the body to a neutral state. Over time, especially in modern-day life, our bodies build up a positive charge due to indoor living, wearing rubber-soled shoes, and our disconnection from Earth and nature. Many of us can go years without directly touching the Earth at all, even if we're outside. In a similar way, when we visit the seaside or natural waterfalls, we absorb the negative ions they produce. Which, unlike their name suggests, are extremely positive and health-creating for the body and mind.

So 'Earthing', then, requires direct contact where the skin touches the soil, sand, water or a conductive surface that is in contact with the Earth. Grounding does not require direct contact but can be achieved through visualisation and imagery, focus and attention. Please do not be alarmed if you feel a sense of being pulled downward, warmth, tingling or any other sensation when grounding. It is your body's way of neutralising any negative energy and bringing balance to your energy. While you do need your conscious mind to instigate the technique of 'grounding', please know that it is not a mental process; rather, it is a natural symbiotic exchange. As you send your energy down, you are allowing energy to come up; you are not simply disposing of your negative energy into the earth. For a long time, I would try to direct, force and push my imagined roots down with my mind and my will, which is a very masculine way of doing something. The feminine energy, which is ultimately what we are trying to connect to here via Mother Earth to foster a deeper connection to our own feminine energy, requires allowing, non-resistance and surrender.

However, when connecting with your Hara centre (your seat of chi/ki) through Hara Breathing, you are actually centring your focus and your energy, thus indirectly grounding, because at the Hara you connect to all that is: the universe inside of yourself.

 Top Tips

* Spend plenty of time outside and surrounded by nature.
* Go barefoot on earth where possible, but please ensure your personal safety by checking for sharp objects or chemicals around that could cause you injury or harm.
* To ground your energy deeply, visualise your feet with roots, much like a tree has, that grow across and penetrate down through the layers of the Earth, connecting right to the centre of the planet at its molten core.
* Keep some house plants to help create a green space within your home.
* Keep an indoor/outdoor water feature to help increase negative ions in the atmosphere.

Keeping a Journal

Journaling is a written record of your thoughts and feelings around your life events. There is nothing fancy about journaling, and it need not be expensive or too time-consuming. My journal actually became my best friend during my mental illness, and I would encourage everyone to keep one. Mine was a spare book I already had lying around from the pound store. I initially kept the book handy for performing my distraction techniques where I would write lists of things I could see when I felt the onset of dissociation and depersonalisation. I also used it to keep a record of my symptoms and would categorise them into three distinct areas: physical sensations, thoughts and my reaction or behaviour—I guess to help me rationalise them. Here is one of my lists taken from my journal at the onset of my PTSD:

Physical Body Symptoms	Cognitive or Thinking Symptoms	Behavioural Reactions
My body is dissolving	I'm going to die	Urge to move from my environment
Light-headedness	There's something wrong with me	Urge to sit down
Tremor / tremble of muscles	I'm going to collapse	Urge to cling to something stable
Superfast thoughts	Am I going mad?	Frantic tidying and sorting things
Detached from my surroundings	I'm dying	More panic

It's really interesting to actually look back at my journal and see how, although my physical body symptoms didn't change (well, perhaps they became less severe), my cognitive/thinking symptoms and behaviours became actions not reactions. This list is taken from my journal some weeks later:

Physical Body Symptoms	Cognitive or Thinking Symptoms	Behavioural Reactions
My body is dissolving	Oh no, not this feeling again	Touch my feet, pat my body
Light-headedness	Ok... I need to change my breathing	Clasp hands over my mouth
Tremor / tremble of muscles	It's ok, I can release this	Shake my body ... move my body
Superfast thoughts	Speak more slowly	Take deep breaths... Hara breathing
Detached from my surroundings	I'm real, I'm alive, this will pass	Visualise myself in a toilet tube!

Over time, however, I began using my journal to write a daily plan, by which time I had been off work for six weeks and felt I needed some structure to my day to aid in my recovery. This probably sounds ridiculous to most people, to have to make a list to remind you to take a shower or to eat dinner, but when you severely lose touch with reality, all normal daily functioning goes out the window. This is also known as Activities of Daily Living (ADL) by the healthcare profession. This then naturally progressed into writing for me, at first about whether I'd managed to adhere to my daily activities then to how I was feeling. Simple stuff like whether I'd had a good day, a bad day. I wrote about my sleeping patterns (or lack of them) and what I was eating. I began to write about all my scary and weird symptoms and used it to keep a record of my dreams, which were off-the-Richter-scale weird during this time. They were extremely intense and vivid, often carrying messages to aid in my recovery.

Over time, my journal became like an addiction. I couldn't go a day without writing. It was a place where I could offload all my inner turmoil without the fear of being judged, without the fear of worrying my loved ones even more than what they were already. You see, as an empath, even when I was so mentally ill, I was still worried about everyone else and, in a sense, trying to protect them. At first, I censored my writing, not divulging my deepest thoughts, worries and problems, but the more I wrote, the harder it became to not fully unleash my inner world onto the paper. Any negative thoughts I had, especially those of an irrational and compulsive nature, those reoccurring thoughts that just wouldn't go away, I began to share, no matter how stupid, scary or dark they seemed. I began to write them all down. At first I ran from the thoughts, not wanting to acknowledge them, trying to avoid them, which only led to further empower them. Then, one afternoon, I was sat crying, scared of who I was becoming, pleading with the universe to make my strange symptoms go away, and I was shown a vision of a vinyl record jumping. The record had a deep scratch etched into the vinyl which kept the needle stuck in one place on a loop of repeat. The rest of the record was fine—in pristine condition, actually; there was just this one area that needed repair. As with all visions, it happened in a millisecond, and so much information was instantly known from the pictures, images and symbols that I saw. I knew then that I was being shown an analogy to what was happening with my mind and cognitive processing. There was nothing seriously wrong with my brain—because let's face it, when you experience mental health issues, you convince yourself that you have every fatal illness and life-threatening condition under the Sun! But it was just like a hardware error; my thought processing was slightly malfunctioning. In fact, it would have probably been more troublesome for me to have had a computer hardware problem, as I am such a technophobe! Anyway, as soon as I could see it for what it was, I could begin to rationalise that I wasn't a bad person and that I wasn't losing control of my mind, so slowly but surely the thoughts began to lose their power over me.

The thoughts became less intrusive and eventually less frequent, but more importantly, when they did happen, I began to see them for what they were: a little blip in the hardware which was no cause for concern. Once I could see more clearly, as opposed to being stuck in a flume of thick smoke and fog like I had been for several months, I knew that I could repair this fault.

Part of my resistance to writing my negative reoccurring thoughts was due to my awareness of the Law of Attraction. For a time when I was not able to think and process information efficiently, I worried that if I actually wrote those thoughts down in black and white, I would somehow be creating them, bringing them into form so into physical manifestation, but in fact, quite the opposite is true. What we resist persists. The negative thoughts held more power when they were constantly being reactivated and re-energised with the emotion of fear when held in the mind and field of my consciousness which surrounds my physical body. Once the thought was released via the spoken word or written, both of which are actions, in effect I was transmuting the energy in that moment. I was bringing it into form so I didn't have to worry about it manifesting at a later date. This way, I became the alchemist and transformed it. That's where our power lies, but it is a conscious choice to take action.

☼ Top Tips

* The journal is only for you, so don't worry about spelling, punctuation or the readability of the writing.
* Write anything... the good, the bad and the ugly.
* Use it to monitor your symptoms: physical, mental, behavioural.
* If you don't like using pen to paper, type it. Use your laptop or your phone. You could even use the voice recorder on your phone if you are more auditory.
* Try to journal as often as you can. Build a habit.
* Don't be afraid to ask questions, too. You will be surprised how easily the answers will come. Perhaps not with a bolt of lightning from the heavens, but in the form of synchronicities and random-chance events... or that's how they may seem at first, but nothing is random.
* Writing your thoughts and worries allows an outlet for your inner world.
* Try to be kind to yourself and non-judgmental in what you uncover about yourself from writing.
* Over time, you may notice particular reoccurring themes in your writing. When you feel stable and able to contemplate this further, explore the patterns, for they will shed light and insight onto your conditioned behaviours and reactions. The shining light of awareness is sometimes all that is needed for transformation to take place.
* You are welcome to download the free Mastering My Crown; Self Discovery Journal, which I created to complement this book.

The Benefits of Physical Activity and Exercising

Physical activity is probably the cheapest miracle cure there is for the prevention and treatment of many diseases.

It is medically proven that physical activity can lower the risk of cardiovascular disease, type 2 diabetes, hip fracture, osteoarthritis, some cancers, depression, dementia and even premature death. Other benefits of exercise and being active include reduced stress, increased self-confidence, weight control, increased feelings of well-being, stronger bones and muscles, increased flexibility/mobility and positive social well-being. Although most people are aware of the benefits of physical activity and exercise on health, the vast majority don't actually meet the current UK government guideline of 150 minutes of moderate aerobic activity every week (for adults aged 19-64). Although it may initially seem a lot, this can be broken down into the more manageable five lots of 30 minutes a week, and even further into two 15-minute brisk walks five days a week. Moderate aerobic activity could include dancing, vigorous gardening or cycling to work, so don't think you have to join a gym to become active! Anything that raises your heart rate, gets you breathing a little faster and feeling warmer will suffice! If you prefer to reduce the duration, you could always increase the intensity to 75 minutes of vigorous physical activity instead broken down into three 25-minute sessions. This could include increasing your effort from walking to jogging/running, aerobics, spinning, sports or walking up inclines such as stairs or hills/mountains if you prefer the outdoors. Also, as we age, we lose muscle mass and strength so guidelines recommend performing two strength-based sessions a week as well. This could simply include performing four functional movements such as standing squats, press-ups against the wall, laying glute bridges and some sit-ups, modified if needed. It doesn't have to be complex or time-consuming, and you certainly don't need any fancy equipment.

Exercise is particularly beneficial to those who suffer from anxiety and panic, because it helps to use up all the stress hormones that have been released due to the fear/stress response. Equally, those suffering from grief and depression would also benefit, because after about 20 minutes of more intense aerobic exercise, your body begins to release neurochemicals called endorphins. These are the body's natural pain reliever that not only act as a sedative but also elevate mood. One kind known as a beta-endorphin is even stronger than morphine! Exercise also stimulates the release of dopamine, our 'pleasure/reward' hormone, and serotonin, our 'happiness hormone', which also helps to regulate mood, sleep and our digestion.

Although exercise and movement is undoubtedly one of the best things you can do for your physical and mental health, rest, recovery and stillness are equally as important. I've been active pretty much my whole life, since my teenage years of playing sports and going to the gym to now at the age of forty finding a love of sea swimming. When I became mentally ill, however, I needed to completely stop and be stationary. Without knowing it, I had come to find being still very difficult, and if I hadn't had a productive day or week, I saw it as time wasted. I guess I also used exercise like a drug, and most drugs simply mask and repress symptoms so we never really get to the root cause of the problem. About four weeks after the onset of my PTSD, my dad would pick me up to take me out for fresh air. Some days I could get out of the car, some days I couldn't. My dad took my arm when I needed stability and support to even walk a few steps initially, but over time we started to take longer walks, eventually building up to eight miles. But then I slipped down the stairs at home, severely bruising my ribs. This developed into costochondritis (inflammation of the cartilage at the sternum and ribs) which causes the most excruciating chest and back pain. Exactly what you don't want when suffering from PTSD and panic attacks—but ironically, exactly what I needed! Although it was a very tough time, my go-to response, which was to flee, move—albeit walk now and not run—began to cause me physical pain. It was at this point I learned to sit in the panic and not run from fear because I physically couldn't due to the pain. Meditation and exercise had always been my means of balancing myself, and now I couldn't do either. This is when I really began to learn about myself; this is when I faced my shadow-self... all the pain, guilt, hurt, resentment, bitterness and grief I held within. I had nowhere to run, nowhere to hide, nowhere to escape to... all I could do was surrender into it all and allow the 'Letting Go' process to unfold.

So while I am an absolute advocate for physical activity and exercise, just be mindful of how and why you exercise the way you do, if you do at all. On the flip side, you might loathe exercise, not wanting to exert yourself, or you may use it as a form of punishment because you 'body shame' or dislike your appearance. Perhaps you want to exercise but lack the motivation and the will; maybe you genuinely don't enjoy moving your body. Everyone is different. I've been an exercise instructor since I was nineteen years old, and the reasons people chose not to exercise or be physically active are varied and complex: lack of time, lack of will, lack of confidence and self-esteem, medical conditions and illnesses, lack of finances, past negative experiences... the list goes on. I suggest really exploring your inner thoughts and feelings regarding your physical activity and exercise habits. Were your parents sporty? Did you get laughed at in school PE because you were no good? Perhaps you've always really wanted to try an activity but feel too self-conscious to give it a go? Whatever the reason, you can change your beliefs and your behaviour. While exercise and physical activity are good, I would say movement is even more crucial. Any movement—smile, stretch, sway, shake, dance, walk, skip or step. Just get into your body... feel it, embrace being alive and having a body, even if it does creak or feel heavy.

A lot of people exercise in a somewhat automated fashion, often following an instructor who tells them exactly how to move their body. Even with more somatic exercise techniques such as yoga and Pilates, I've seen many people fail to consciously connect to their body. The most profound technique I have ever used, which really helps to open up the communication with your body, becoming more aware of your inner experience, is Self-Myofascial Release (SMR). This uses equipment such as foam rollers and stimulation/massage balls to help release chronic tightness within muscle bands and of the myofascia. 'Myo' means muscle, and 'fascia' is the system of web-like connective tissue that permeates the whole body. It's the closest thing to having a massage you can do alone, and I believe it was this somatic exercise technique that really assisted my body through the healing and recovery process after my mental illness. Just be careful searching for stimulation or massage balls on Google if you intend to buy any—I can't promise what will come up!

As my body and mental state began improving, I began to suffer from extreme periods of fatigue where my body would just ache from head to toe. Even my fingers and bones would ache, and I couldn't understand why because I hadn't exerted myself. I would also have these really bad flares-up of chest and upper-back pain, which I knew was costochondritis but later came to realise was repressed emotional pain too, but I do wonder whether I had fibromyalgia, which I know can be a secondary condition to anxiety and PTSD. However, because of my training in exercising special populations with medical conditions, I knew I needed to heal my body in stages: first the myofascial tissue and muscles through SMR and gentle stretching. Then I could progress to more cardiovascular exercise but only in the form of very low-intensity walking. The minute my heart rate went above 50-60% of my maximum heart rate for my age (90-110 beats per minute), instead of feeling the positive effects of exercise, I would feel completely wiped out for days. It was such a learning curve having to re-introduce my body to exercise in this way, and I learnt to be much gentler with myself. Finally, about a year after my initial PTSD, I was able to progress to longer low-intensity cardiovascular exercise such as jogging and stationary cycling. Strength training came last. Even now, some four years later, I can only manage lower levels of resistance, so I have stuck to bodyweight resistance training methods such as Pilates, yoga and suspension training rather than lifting actual weights.

 Top Tips

* Just MOVE! Movement is so important to keep the lymphatic fluid moving, our blood and oxygen circulating and to prevent our energy within our meridians from stagnating.
* Find an activity that you enjoy... stretching, yoga, Pilates, tai chi, dancing, walking, biking, gardening, skipping, hiking, swimming, playing, etc.
* Use a buddy scheme. Find someone who you can be active with, so you can motivate each other.
* Use a pedometer or smartwatch to keep track of your steps.
* Scout through YouTube. There are so many great free channels and exercise workouts. Just choose your instructor wisely.
* Set yourself realistic targets to meet your exercise goals. Not only will this boost your confidence, but it will also boost your dopamine levels from accomplishing a task!
* Be willing to adapt and change how you exercise to suit your current level of ability and fitness.
* If you find yourself feeling more fatigued after exercising, use the very basic and well-known age predicted formula to check you are not exceeding your maximum heart rate. To work it out, simply retract your age from 220. Also, if you have experienced recent trauma and have an over-sensitised nervous system, you may find that exercising at 50% of your maximum heart rate is more suitable. To do this, however, you will require some form of heart rate monitor or smartwatch.
* Try some somatic-based exercise. I currently teach an online 'Mastering Me' Body Class that teaches you how to honour and heal your physical body by releasing any tension, stress and trauma. I also taught Trigger Point Pilates™ for over six years, which

I found amazing and uses Pilates-based movements and equipment to release the body (muscles, joints and myofascia). Check out if there is an instructor near you: www.tppilates.com. There are also many other somatic based therapies and forms of exercise out there which may be more suited to you, but at least you now know what to look for.

* If you lack masculine energy, you may find that learning to be more organised is needed. Look at your week ahead and plan in your physical activity/exercise like you would a hair or doctor appointment. However, if you are balancing out your feminine energy like I was, you may need to learn to be more flexible and exercise when your body allows, not when your mind tells you.

Autonomous Sensory Meridian Response (ASMR)

After my panic attacks began to subside, my body and mind were left in a rather numb and bewildered state. That's when insomnia kicked in. Although I became extremely exhausted, my brain just wouldn't allow me to fall to sleep. I would just feel like I was dropping off and then I would literally hear a click, my eyes would shoot open, heart would race and I would feel more alert than I had been during the whole day. It was at this point I came across Autonomous Sensory Meridian Response (ASMR).

Now, I must warn you, it's not for everyone and you have to take the time to discover which type is best for you, if any. At first, it can seem a very strange concept. Probably like many, I initially thought, 'What the hell is this all about?' Anyway, I shall continue, because it did help me, although there is no scientific research to back this up (at least none I am aware of). ASMR is a term coined in 2010 that describes a tingling sensation that originates at the back of the head and travels to the scalp and down the spine. It involves listening to another person whispering or using mundane objects to make gentle soft sounds which can have a relaxing effect. There are now hundreds of videos on YouTube that explore this phenomenon. It is generally unrelated to sexual arousal, although it can occur from such physiological responses. For me, it certainly wasn't a sexual sensation that was invoked, but when I felt alone in the darkness of night, not able to sleep, it used to bring me a sense of comfort. Although my mind at this point still wouldn't allow me to sleep due to my trauma and fear response, listening to ASMR did allow my body space and time to deeply relax, which forms a huge part of the recovery process.

 Top Tips
* Find a video and voice that resonates with you and brings you comfort.
* Sample a few before you decide to actually listen to the full video at bedtime.
* It's not for everyone, but you don't know until you try it.
* You might find listening to a progressive relaxation more suitable. In fact, I often share free audios on my social media.

Sleep Hygiene

We all know how invigorating it feels to wake up from a good night's sleep, but unfortunately, many people don't get the seven to eight hours a night that scientists at the National Sleep Foundation say we need... even without mental illness ($_{17}$). Sleep is essential, just like eating, drinking and breathing. It boosts our immune system, helping to fight infection, and helps our brain function more efficiently so we can think more clearly, memorise better and learn things more easily. It also recalibrates our limbic or emotional brain so our mood is enhanced and we can more positively face the day and any challenges life throws at us.

Our 24-hour sleep-wake cycle consists of approximately 16 hours of wakefulness and eight hours of sleep and is influenced by our circadian rhythm, environmental factors and the amount of time spent awake (sleep pressure). The circadian rhythm, the body's natural internal clock that carries out many biological functions and processes over a 24-hour cycle is overseen by none other than our commander-in-chief... the hypothalamus. Who, if you remember, is part of the reptilian brain and limbic system responsible for our emotional state, as well as influencing the rise and fall in hormone levels, controlling habits, digestion, body temperature, etc. Well, it is within the hypothalamus that a large bundle of nerves can be found known as the suprachiasmatic nucleus (I prefer the abbreviation of SCN myself), which instructs the pineal gland to produce melatonin—and this, ladies and gentlemen, is the master hormone of sleep! Information about the levels of incoming light from the optic nerves travel from the eyes to the brain, and when there is less light, the SCN tells the brain to make more melatonin, which makes you sleepy. Put simply, the release of melatonin is stimulated by darkness and is reduced by incoming light, so making sure you have adequate darkness in the bedroom is key.

We should also consider our sleep hygiene in trying to foster more restful and healthy sleeping patterns. This includes those behaviours we adopt just before bedtime and more generic lifestyle behaviours such as our exercise levels, alcohol consumption and our eating habits. Although evidence shows that exercise helps to improve sleep quality, vigorous exercise just before bed can inhibit sleep due to an increase in body temperature and a stress hormone surge. Our sleep-wake cycle is also influenced by sleep pressure— that is, the longer we stay awake, the greater our urge to sleep. This growing urge to sleep is said to be influenced by a molecule called adenosine that builds in the bloodstream the longer we stay awake ($_{18}$). During sleep, adenosine is evacuated by the brain, and thus when we wake the sleep pressure becomes low once again, but if you haven't had your full quota of sleep and residual adenosine hasn't been properly processed, you can still feel groggy. This is when many people reach for the hit of caffeine first thing, to stoke the fires and get them going!

I've always been sensitive to caffeine so can't touch it; I've always had blackout blinds and regularly exercised, which may explain why I'd never had problems with my sleep. Even immediately following the onset of my PTSD, surprisingly I was still able to sleep. However, as time progressed, the quality and length of my sleep, and my ability to fall asleep, changed drastically.

Initially, I would have a mild panic attack on waking. I think it was the shock and shift in my realities, since my dream time felt clearer and more real than my waking life. Having a physical body was such a shock to my consciousness and the hypersensitivity too much to bear, so I would dissociate. I always managed to hold onto my physical reality, however. I mean, I always knew I was in my house and I knew I was alive, but it was like my surroundings were slipping away. Like I was getting further away from the world and everything in it. Then, one night, I just couldn't go to sleep. That's when insomnia started. It didn't cause me stress initially, because I would just watch my favourite films I had seen numerous times before to avoid being overstimulated. I thought to myself, 'Well, I'll sleep when I need to,' but then days turned into weeks and weeks turned into months and I started to get frustrated and worried. My eyes would eventually get heavy, I'd get that drop in consciousness for a split second, and then *zap*—it was like having a bolt of lightning hit me, jolting me awake. I became aware of an actual clicking sound in my head... reminded me of the noise my heating makes when it turns on. My husband could see I was getting more distressed and exhausted, so he suggested we have a marathon film night where we would bring the duvet downstairs and not worry about whether we slept or not. It was that night I had a shift in my sleeping behaviour for the better. '*Ahhhh, what a relief...*' I knew I had slept before I had even opened my eyes, and I didn't even care for how long. When I looked at my clock, a whole two hours had past and I was elated, but then I heard my condescending shadow-self say, 'It was the crystal that helped and nothing you did.' I was initially confused because I had actually removed every single crystal that I owned from my house after my Dark Night of the Soul... or so I thought. All my tumbled pieces I used for my healing practice, my decorative pieces and every single piece of jewellery with a mineral or crystal attached was expelled. Due to my incredibly weak emotional and mental state, their vibrations were actually overpowering me and negatively interfering with my own energy, so I transferred them all to my parents' house. So, of course, I instantly disputed my shadow-self's claim, but then I was drawn to a hoodie that I had brought downstairs to wear but had ended up placing on the arm of the sofa instead... where my head had been. I checked the pockets immediately, and there it was: one tiny little stone that I had obviously missed during my earlier crystal cull! It was a little black Apache Tear, and this little beauty had not only eased me out of insomnia but also out of my crystal phobia!

You may have wondered why I haven't suggested the use of crystals to assist with mental illness until now, and that is because every single mineral, although each has generic qualities, will affect people very differently. Crystal Therapy is considered non-invasive, meaning you don't ingest or penetrate the physical body in any way, and most would think then that no harm can come from their use. But you now know that the human body has its own crystalline matrix, just like a mineral or crystal does, and interaction between two can cause changes at the most fundamental and cellular level. Unlike quartz which is piezoelectric—which, if you remember, means it emits a constant regular pulse and can be programmed—an Apache Tear is amorphous. This means it is not crystalline and doesn't have a consistent internal structure or lattice. It is actually a volcanic glass, not a mineral, and energetically it constricts, contains and protects, which is great for someone who can't sleep due to expanded energy or, in the case of severe trauma, a completely blown crown chakra and dysfunctional limbic system. It is also one of the gentler crystals used for assisting in the release of grief from the emotional body. Again, use your own discernment and intuition as to whether an Apache Tear would be suitable for you.

In summary, sleep and health are strongly related and poor sleep and mental illness can go hand in hand. While stress, anxiety and panic disorders tend to reduce the ability to sleep, depression can cause the opposite problem whereby the need for sleep is greatly increased. Either way, applying some of the top tips listed below can help improve the duration, quality and timing of your sleep.

 Top Tips

* Develop a bedtime routine if possible.
* Ensure there is adequate darkness... remember, melatonin, our sleep hormone, is stimulated by darkness! Maybe invest in some black-out blinds.
* Limit watching TV before bed as it can stimulate the mind and nervous system.
* Limit LED and screen time, reducing your exposure to 'blue light'.
* Ensure the bedroom is of a comfortable temperature with limited noise.
* Avoid eating spicy or heavy meals for two to three hours before bed so your digestive system is not overburdened and the body is able to do its job of rest, repair and restore.
* Avoid strenuous exercise for two to three hours before you wish to sleep to avoid any stress-hormone surge.
* Check out your 'chronotype' which is your genetic sleep predisposition connected to your PER3 gene. Go online and complete the Morning-Eveningness Questionnaire at www.sleepfoundation.org, which confirms if you are a 'Morning Lark' or 'Night Owl'.
* Keep your journal handy to write down your ruminating thoughts, worries or things you need to remember that pop into your mind when you become still.
* Keep a dream journal to see if your subconscious is trying to get your attention.

* Use the 8 Step Sequence as a night-time ritual to help reset your physical body, leading to a more balanced limbic system, which is ultimately responsible for your sleep-wake cycle.
* If you have nocturnal panic attacks, avoid remaining in bed and riding it out. Get up and shake your body, move, stretch, then reset your physical body using the remaining steps of the 8 Step Sequence.
* Consider acquiring an Apache Tear, but be sure to cleanse it regularly with running water and sunlight.

Keeping Hydrated and Eating Well

I will start with hydration since the human body can survive longer without food than water. Although figures suggest that the body consists of 60-70% water, it's more like 50-60%, in my experience of measuring hydration as a Health and Well-being Advisor. Most people know they should drink plenty of water, but many don't actually know how much or why. There are mixed views regarding suggested levels of water consumption for health, with American research recommending 8x8 (eight glasses of eight ounces of fluid per day) compared with the UK guideline of six to eight glasses a day (equivalent to 1.2 litres). In warmer temperatures and if you are physically active or when you exercise, you should consume more. Water within the body helps to flush away waste, aiding the digestive system and evacuation of the bowels; it stabilises body temperature and it cushions the brain and spinal cord. Just becoming mildly dehydrated could impair mental functioning, resulting in poorer memory, concentration and focus.

The myofascia within the body also needs to be sufficiently hydrated in order to do its job properly. That is to attach, stabilise, enclose and separate every muscle and internal organ within the body, acting as a connector and link between the bones, ligaments, tendons, muscles, arteries, veins, nerves and even our skin. When myofascial tissue becomes dehydrated, it loses its ability to slide and flow, resulting in sticky tissue and limited mobility. In terms of anxiety and fear—remember how the body increases the heart rate to get the blood and therefore oxygen around the body quicker? Well, this raises the blood pressure. That's the pressure in the arteries during the contraction phase of the heartbeat (the systolic higher figure) and the pressure in the arteries during the relaxation phase of the heartbeat (the diastolic lower figure). Since blood is more than 90% water, when you are dehydrated, blood volume levels drop, which temporally increases your blood pressure, so by being dehydrated you are also putting the heart under undue strain. To manage anxiety and fear means needing to self-regulate to bring the body back to homeostasis or balance, so ensuring that the body has enough fluid helps this process. I am very lucky—I actually love water—but many people don't, so I suggest finding an alternative such as weak squash, herbal teas or flavoured water. If you choose fruit juices, just be mindful of the high sugar content, especially if you suffer from diabetes or metabolic syndrome. Any caffeinated drinks, such as coffee, energy drinks and alcohol, can have a diuretic effect on the body, meaning it helps eliminate salt (sodium) and water. So if you can't function in the morning without a hit of your favourite coffee, ask yourself: why? Did you need it because you have a dysfunctional sleep-wake cycle? Is it habit? Do you simply like the taste? Either way, just be mindful that caffeine can exacerbate anxiety and an already over-stimulated nervous system.

I remember meditating some years ago (before my mental illness) and pondering what I needed to do to clear a foggy head I was experiencing, and my intuition said, 'You need to drink a gallon of still water.' A rather normal insight and request compared to my usual intel, so off I went and bought some. After I finished it over the course of 24 hours, I thought to myself... 'I should continue with this... It must be healthier.' Not the amount, I must add—the drinking bottled water part. But after about two weeks, I started to get an upset stomach, I felt exhausted and could feel something depleting within me. I started to contemplate why I felt so awful so asked my spirit guide... 'Too much bottled water!' he said.

Defensively, I quickly retaliated with, 'But I felt guided to drink it!'

His response: 'Your intuition guided you to drink a gallon of still water.'

Slightly annoyed with myself, I realised how my mind and ego had assumed what was best for me. My assumption that bottled water must be healthier was a belief perhaps from advertising or from what I had been told sometime in the distant past, but the fact was, it wasn't. At this point I realised the delicacy and fine balance that my body needs to keep me balanced—after all, not all water is the same. There are minute differences in trace elements, minerals and the general hardness of any given water. What can bring balance in one day can cause imbalance over several days. So yet again my lesson was this... to listen to my body and listen to my intuition with accuracy and not to what my mind thinks! If you are sensitive physically, emotionally and energetically, my advice is: always check in with yourself. Don't be fooled by your habit-creating conscious mind; your intuition and gut feeling know best... if you bother to check, that is!

If you really want to power-up your drinking water, you could always bless it, programme it or infuse it with positive words! You may have heard of Dr Masaru Emoto, a Japanese researcher and alternative healer who in 2006 scientifically proved that thoughts and intentions can alter physical reality ($_{19}$). His study involved a group of approximately 2000 people in Tokyo reciting a prayer of gratitude towards samples of water over 5,000 miles away in an electromagnetically shielded room in California. The results proved that positive intentions produced symmetrical, well-formed and aesthetically pleasing ice crystals from the water in question. If you haven't seen the pictures, I really do recommend having a look... he also did similar experiments involving rice. Given that the human body is comprised of such high levels of water, just imagine what effect our consciousness in the form of repetitive thoughts and beliefs has on our bodies. Which is all the more reason to harness our unique gift of being able to speak the spoken word... to create health, love and positive vibrations. It was Archangel Zadkiel that once told me 'the spoken word creates', so don't underestimate the power of your words.

You might be surprised to find that I am not going to discuss nutrition in any great detail because one person's cure is another person's poison where food is concerned. One style of eating can be health promoting for you, while it could completely disrupt the fine balance of vitamins, minerals and micronutrients within another. Plus, eating and dietary habits are highly personal, and I am in no position to tell anyone what and how to eat. Again, I say: use your intuition in making food choices, and just like the seasons change, so does what our body requires. A balanced diet, however, should consist of a mixture of proteins, carbohydrates, fats, vitamins and minerals, including fresh fruit, vegetables and fibre. How and in what form you consume them is for only you to decide.

During my PTSD, I wasn't eating a great deal, and when I did, whatever I consumed gave me a great deal of gas. Remember, during even mild stress or anxiety, blood flow to the digestive organs is inhibited due to the 'fight or flight' response redistributing the blood to the muscles and other organs that are needed to fight or flee. So I do suggest eating little and often to not overburden your already overworked digestive system, plus this will keep blood sugars stabilised. Even before my mental illness, I had a sensitive gut, and even foods that are considered 'healthy' such as certain fruits and vegetables are a big no-go for me. You may find keeping a food diary helpful to monitor how you feel after eating, and as simple as this sounds, if you feel light, energised and nourished, it was probably what your body needed. If you feel heavy, bloated and tired afterwards, it probably wasn't. Also, processed foods not only have low nutrient value but also have pretty much zero good chi! That also goes for any foods you nuke... I mean microwave! I'm going to keep it real here... although I eat pretty healthily, my diet and nutritional habits could be a lot better, but I am human and find being disciplined with food the hardest of all areas to maintain.

⚡ Top Tips

* Keep hydration a priority in managing your health.
* If you don't like water, find a fluid that you do like (unfortunately I don't mean of the alcoholic variety).
* If your problem lies in forgetting to drink, try setting some reminders on your phone or purchase these cool bottles that tell you how much you should have consumed by a certain time of day.
* Consider a glass, stainless steel or copper reusable water bottle or container instead of plastic, which can contain bisphenol A (or BPA for short) which is an endocrine disruptor. You don't want to waste all that good time you've spent regulating your body and hormones in the 8 Step Sequence, plus reusable alternatives are much kinder to our planet... Mother Earth!
* Reduce your caffeine intake if needed, perhaps swapping to decaf or herbal varieties instead.
* Bless, programme or infuse your drinking water with positive energy.

Flower Essences

Flower essences are a form of alternative medicine that use the vibrational and energy signature of a plant or flower to help balance negative emotions within the body. I was sceptical at first, but when I began using them, I was pleasantly surprised by their immediate yet gentle effect. Being extremely sensitive to toxins and medications, they offered me support when I felt I had limited options. Although flowers and herbs have been used for medicinal purposes for centuries, it was Dr Edward Bach from England who first developed the system of flower and plant-based essences. Although he was trained in conventional medicine, he came to believe that illness arose from a disharmony between the body and mind and that emotional well-being was the key to health. Dr Bach spent his later years studying the healing properties of various plants and flowers and their effects on human emotions. He created 38 different flower remedies by the time of his death in 1936, including the very well-known 'Rescue Remedy'. This is the first flower essence I ever used, and it really did help to ease my feelings of fear and panic. Interestingly, I was guided to buy it about two weeks before I had my Dark Night of the Soul, but due to being stuck in extreme fear, I didn't actually take it until a few weeks after. Had I known of their powerful yet gentle effect, I would have started using them long ago.

The flower essences come in tiny dropper bottles that hold extreme dilutions of the flower's essence in a solution of water and brandy. Most brands that sell them offer consultations or questionnaires to help you decipher which flower essences are right for you at a particular time. I never paid for any consultation, however, and just used my intuition when buying them.

I have accumulated a whole range of flower essences from varying brands over the last few years... yet another healing tool to add to my bag. I now use them as and when I feel called to. Mother Earth really is the panacea for all ills.

 Top Tips
 * Bach flower remedies are not the only brand of flower essences available, and I suggest doing your own research and letting your intuition guide you to a brand and essence that feels right for you.
 * Word of caution... Flower essences can contain anywhere from 25-40% brandy in the solution, so if you are recovering from alcoholism, I strongly suggest against using them.

Getting Creative
Due to the coronavirus and strict lockdown measures we have seen much of the arts industry taken away, all live gigs, music concerts, theatre shows and ballets stopped, and museums, art galleries and other cultural institutions

closed. Not only have performers lost their income but many have become isolated and unable to maintain their technical and artistic skills, bringing added worry on top of job insecurities and financial strain. Meanwhile, the countless people who would visit and enjoy such artistic expressions have also been deprived of such beauty, inspiration, fun and social interaction. As you now understand, it is important to allow the body and mind to express itself, not only to use up the hormones produced within the body but to transform the emotions and energy that anxiety, fear, loss or grief can create. Taking part in creative activities creates a sense of joy, fulfilment, relaxation and increased feelings of well-being and can include anything from gardening to baking, painting to doodling, singing to dancing. Some will simply see such activities as hobbies, while for others they may be a profession or career, but when used as means of therapy, they really help us tap into our non-exhaustive creative potential. Such activities have therapeutic and stress-busting qualities to them because we immerse ourselves fully into the activity at hand, time ceases to exist and our conscious mind has a rest.

Art therapy is a well-established form of psychotherapy that has been around for over 70 years, and the emergence of adult colouring books in the last couple of years is a simple way to tap into the wonderful therapeutic effects of art. When I was housebound with PTSD, I created cards for birthdays and special occasions, but I soon got bored as I found the need to be so precise and detailed limiting. Usually, attention to detail was something I would thrive on, but I now found it incredibly frustrating and tiring, so I stopped. Before my mental illness, I had created angelic art, where I would simply sit with a blank canvas and allow whatever angel wanted to be known to manifest through me and out onto the canvas. However, this involved opening my energy field, something I was now too scared to do; plus I was frozen in fear, which was actually blocking my inspiration. Therefore, I had to find a different way to be creative. I had to learn to tap into my own divine creative force within and not rely on any other for my inspiration. This alone felt very daunting at first. I knew

I was harbouring something very dark within, and I was too scared to unleash my inner world onto paper or canvas in fear of what I would see.

It was at this point I discovered a technique called Neurographic art, which stems from the original method called Neurographica, developed by a Russian psychologist and entrepreneur in 2014. 'Neuro' means brain and 'graphic' means image, and the process basically involves drawing free-flowing, irregular and non-patterned lines onto paper. The lines should overlap but not be of a consistent or meaningful pattern, thus representing the chaos of negative emotions and thoughts within. You then begin to transform the lines (your inner conflicts) by curving them out. Every time the lines meet, creating a sharp corner, you soften and curve it out with your pen/marker and then colour in the patterns and shapes that you have created. I am no expert in this area but wanted to acknowledge its existence as I found it helpful. It gave me some parameters to work within that felt safe, and this method enabled me to start opening up that creative block, letting that energy out of my body. It felt good, especially as I didn't have to think... I couldn't do anything that involved thinking or using my conscious mind at that time—my neocortex was well and truly offline! If I did do anything that needed brain power, I got very cloudy, overwhelmed and even more exhausted than I already was. I have given a somewhat simplistic view of the process here just so you can get a feel for what it involves, but should you feel compelled, you could research it further.

I then began a beginner's art course delivered by my fabulous cousin Kerrie, so I felt comfortable and safe to attend. It was during this time I attempted a technique called fluid art which was extremely fun but very messy, and it was at this point 'EmMe Arts' was born. I'm still experimenting, playing and having fun developing a style but am loving the feeling of freedom being creative gives me.

It was my forty-first birthday, during the early days of our first lockdown here in Wales, and instead of gifts, I gave my group of friends the challenge of recreating a photo of us all in any medium and style they wished. It was so wonderful to see everyone's take and different interpretations of the same photo, but what made me giggle more was seeing my 'uncreative friends' out of their comfort zones. The friends (and you know who you are) who had always proclaimed 'I haven't got a creative bone in my body' proved themselves wrong. They also told me how they secretly enjoyed getting their creative hat on, so to speak—so you can too. I challenge you now—just start.

Top Tips

* Find a creative outlet for your thoughts and emotions (which are really just energy in motion).
* Examples include: gardening, flower potting, arts and crafts, drawing, doodling, painting, felting, playing a musical instrument, dancing, knitting, sewing, baking, photography, dancing, pottery, quilting, poetry, writing, creating a blog or YouTube channel.
* If finance is an issue for you, try to use household items that you already have, upcycling old items and giving them a new lease of life.
* Be willing to feel like a complete beginner (or 'utter crap', as my ego told me so many times) but do it anyway.
* Everyone has creative potential within! Yes, everyone... even you! You reading this, who has already begun to wince at the thought of being creative and can't wait to get on to the next chapter.
* Learn to play and experiment with being creative and tap into your childlike innocence and wonder again.
* Remember, you are doing this for you and no one else. No external permission is needed.
* Remember, when you adopt a creative method of expression, this will help to keep your energy flowing, particularly your sacral chakra.
* Enjoy the process. It's not a test or a competition.

Making Lasting Behaviour Change
In exercise psychology, there is a model known as the Stages of Behaviour Change which puts people on a scale of how ready they are to adopt a different behaviour. The stages of

behaviour change are: pre-contemplation, contemplation, preparation, action, maintenance and relapse. The fact that you are even reading this book means that you are already contemplating change and are aware that things could be improved in your life. Hopefully, if you follow the advice in this book, you will move through the preparation stage with ease and be ready to take action. Taking action, however—any action requires effort, and applying the techniques within this book are no exception. Maintaining that action requires continued effort over time, which is commitment and discipline. Just remember that with any behaviour change, there may come a time when you relapse. Maybe your motivation will dwindle, perhaps you will simply forget to perform the 8 Step Sequence or won't bother to write your 'Letting Go' letters. You might even think, 'What's the point?' Just know that this is normal, and the key is to not berate yourself for it. So many times I've seen people who haven't stuck to a healthy lifestyle choice say, 'Well I've messed up now, so I might as well quit.' Or they miss a few exercise sessions or meditation practice and say, 'I've fallen off the wagon now,' so binge on fast food, crisps, chocolate or whatever their self-soothing behaviour of choice is. It's ok not to be perfect all the time, but the most important thing is... you don't give up! It's ok to give up temporarily—maybe you have some more preparation to do, or maybe you just needed to be still a little longer. Perhaps you need to spend time witnessing yourself, getting to know yourself and how you behave when you have a tough, tiring week or when things don't go your way. See it as an opportunity for learning about yourself. The key lies in fully accepting exactly where you now find yourself and forgiving yourself for any way that you may have disappointed yourself.

Know that it is ok to fail but that the real growth comes from the strength and courage it takes to always get back up. In doing so you will come to realise just how powerful you are. Remember, the only constant is change, and although you may feel like you have been stuck in a particular emotional state for a long time, it will pass. It might pass like a kidney stone... but it will pass! When I went on my first ever skiing trip, I didn't have lessons because I like to learn more experimentally and I was with a friend who was an expert skier and patient teacher. I fell over so many times, but I just kept getting back up. When I hated myself for who I had become after my PTSD, no longer the independent and positive person who I had always been, I practised radical self-forgiveness. Over and over, forgiving myself for any ways in which I felt I had failed and forgiving myself for anything I wasn't ready to forgive myself for! It is certainly the road less travelled but always so worth it. In an age where so much information is at our fingertips—although this is a wonderful gift—there is a tendency for people to think that because they have read about a topic, that qualifies them to be considered an expert in a particular area. While I am all for education and continued learning and understand that knowledge is power—doing, taking action, practice and repetition hold greater power. Doing is the key to self-mastery. Reading the information within this book is great, but following the guidance and actually doing the work is much better. That's the part you need to do alone. I can support you and guide you, but ultimately, with the utmost love in my heart, I say this... With the choices you make, you are the only one who can change and transform yourself.

 Top Tips

* Start with small changes that you can actually achieve. Use the acronym SMART when planning your goals: specific, measurable, attainable, relevant and time bound.
* Regularly revise the goals and expectations you have for yourself. Remember you can only do your best at any given moment, and your best will always change.
* Be willing to fail.
* Allow yourself to actually do nothing sometimes. Rest and stillness are a very much-needed part of the growth process. Evolving, shifting your consciousness and transforming your inner world require periods of both action and non-action.
* Self-mastery comes from knowing when to push and when to pause, and we won't always get that right.
* Practise radical self-forgiveness.

CHAPTER 13

The Bigger Picture

What Has Astrology Got to Do with Anxiety, Fear, Loss and Grief?
I wanted to share with you the bigger picture of what is
unfolding in our world today to perhaps shift your vantage
point and enable you to see things from a different
perspective. Once you uncover the truth that everything
is energy with a unique vibration and frequency and that
everything in the entire universe is connected, you will begin to
realise that what goes on in the outer world around you is
also going on within you... your inner world.

This therefore brings me to the topic of astrology. I
understand that your initial thoughts may be, 'What on
earth has astrology got to do with anxiety, fear, loss and
grief?' But you see, it has everything to do with it, and I
would be doing you a huge disservice if I failed to mention
it. If, however, you've read your stars or horoscopes in a
newspaper or magazine and have disregarded the whole
idea, I don't blame you. That—what's known as Sun sign
astrology—is like looking at one tiny grain of sand on a vast
stretch of beach. Although important, it is only a minute part
of a much larger, complex and intricate study of how the
planets weave a magical dance—or what Pythagoras called
'the harmony of the spheres'—which sets the tone for each
of us individually but also for our world collectively.

On the 20th January 2020, two planets came together in our
skies unleashing a whole new wave of energy into the ether,
one that had been building since 2018. An energy so powerful

that our world as we knew it would change forever. The first known recorded case of the coronavirus in the UK was on 31st January 2020, and while some might say the relatively close timing of both events is just a coincidence, don't pass judgement just yet. To understand the true magnitude of such a planetary meeting, you need to at least grasp the basics of Western astrology, which puts the twelve signs of the zodiac (Aries, Taurus, Gemini, Cancer, Leo, Virgo, Libra, Scorpio, Sagittarius, Capricorn, Aquarius and Pisces) in the sky around the Earth, and split into 30 degree segments. It's helpful to think of an orange... each segment would represent a zodiac sign with the core being where Earth is located. Each zodiac sign carries a particular quality to it and can be broken down further into one of the four elements (fire, earth, air and water). Each planet then has like its very own personality, or what's known as its 'archetype', with a particular frequency of energy.

At the exact moment you were born, all the planets and other celestial bodies were in different parts of the sky and in different zodiac signs, which are reflected in your natal birth chart, underpinning your very unique personality and energies that you embody in this life. The planets don't stop moving at this moment, however; they continue to spiral through space and around the zodiac, creating different energies that can be felt here on Earth.

The Saturn and Pluto Meeting
The two planets that came together (also known as a conjunction in astrology) on the 20th January 2020 were Pluto and Saturn, and their merged energy was felt viscerally throughout the whole world that year. They are two of the very slowly moving outer planets within our solar system and, as such, their effects build over time. Pluto moved into the zodiac sign of Capricorn in 2008 and Saturn later in 2017, and they finally meet up with each other at 22 degrees of Capricorn on 20th January 2020. Although this meeting happens approximately every 36 years, the last time they

met in Capricorn was in 1518, the year the monk and priest Martin Luther's 95 theses became the seed that would birth the Protestant Reformation of the Catholic Church!

Pluto, known as Lord of the Underworld in Roman Mythology, is closely tied to the Ancient Greek God Hades and represents death, transformation and renewal. Pluto personifies ultimate power... the primordial energy of instinct and our life force energy rising to procreate, so also rules biologically the processes of sex and birth too. Just as a diamond is formed deep within the Earth's mantle from a powerful transformation caused by heat and pressure, we too are transformed by the pressure of Pluto energy. It asks us to delve deep into our own psyche to acknowledge our own personal issues that we might not want to face. However, when we do, what is lurking in the depths, hidden and occulted from view, can be purged and freed in an alchemical transformative process. Power and desire ultimately create greed, lust, jealousy, hatred, revenge, resentment... all the human emotions that are condemned and thought of as evil, so as a result get pushed down into our bodies, into our cells and into our subconscious (our own underworld). As discussed earlier in the book, such rejected parts of ourselves create our 'shadow-selves'—the worst parts of us, the worst parts of humanity.

Exposing the truth of what is hidden and repressed in the shadows is the realm of Scorpio, the zodiac sign ruled by Pluto. This has been the reoccurring theme for so many over the last few years, particularly anyone who has abused their power for personal gain. You could say that the highest expression of Pluto's personality or energy is to decay, dismantle, breakdown and shatter, not purely for the sake of creating misery and destruction but to purify and resurrect through transformation to create a rebirth. Pluto is one of the smallest but farthest planets from Earth and takes 248 years to orbit the Sun, so completes one full cycle of the zodiac in the same time. Therefore, Pluto's energy is generational and has its affect over a long period of time.

Saturn has had a longer and more complex past than Pluto, having evolved through the pantheons, so his exact origins are not clear. Said to have derived from Cronus, the Ancient Greek god of seed, harvest, agriculture and periodical renewal, and later becoming associated with Chronos, god of time to the Romans, Saturn in astrology represents the passing of time, so our past and future, including the lessons we have to learn throughout our lives to reach maturity. Saturn is personified as the strict rule enforcer so constricts and confines teaching responsibility through restriction and firm boundaries. Many people, even those who don't follow astrology, have at least heard of the much-anticipated 'Saturn Return' which happens at around the age of 30 and again at around the age of 60 (plus or minus a few years). This is because Saturn takes 29.5 years to travel around the zodiac, so it is at these ages that Saturn returns to the exact same spot in the zodiac to where it was when you were born. Saturn's return can be felt as a sobering reality check, a time when we are required to grow up and take a deep look at our choices to date that may or may not please us or be in line with our path and destiny. We begin to see time as running away from us and are faced with the prospect of our own mortality. If you live to the ripe old age of 90, you'll be lucky enough to experience a third Saturn Return—and I say lucky, because it means you have been blessed with long years of living! Saturn therefore represents fears too, all the worries and concerns that accompany aging, such as health complaints, age-related diseases and, of course, physical death. It also represents the worries we may face when we are responsible and dutiful adults, such as being able to provide for our families and being respected in our jobs and professions. But Saturn isn't all work and no play. When we show dedication, commitment and perseverance in the face of adversity, we are rewarded with wisdom and see tangible accomplishments physically manifest.

So now you have a little more understanding of the personalities of Pluto and Saturn, let's take a deeper look at Capricorn, where this meeting took place. As previously mentioned, the zodiac signs can be categorised using the four elements—fire, earth, air or water—but they are further split into three different types of energy (called modalities). Cardinal signs are starting/energising energy, fixed signs are doing/stabilising energy, and mutable signs are finishing/flexible energy. Capricorn is a cardinal (starting) earth energy, and when the Sun enters it, marks the start of winter here in the Northern Hemisphere. Capricorn's flavour is earthy and grounded, stoic, practical, disciplined, patient and hardworking. It also represents the physical world of form, the father and the patriarchy, the system of society and government that puts the elder male at the head of such structures, the ones our physical realities have for millennia been based on. Saturn actually rules Capricorn, so is super happy and powerful when travelling through this part of the zodiac. Capricorn is said to rule the skeletal system, knees, joints and teeth too, because they are the very structure of the human body. However, the true essence and highest expression of Capricorn energy is the wise elder who has committed and dedicated their life to fulfilling their true calling and purpose, whatever that may be. Love or loathe the British monarchy, no one can dispute the life-long devotion and duty Queen Elizabeth II has given to her people and country. Interestingly, Her Royal Highness has Saturn right on the career sector of her natal birth chart and Capricorn on the ascendant, the area that represents a person's outlook on life and how they are perceived by others.

So if we piece all of this together, you can start to see that the planetary meeting (conjunction) that took place in January 2020 was a catalyst for the death/transformation (Pluto) of structures (Saturn), particularly those of a patriarchal nature (Capricorn). Pluto's energy is therefore destabilising and deconstructing the very foundation modern society has been built on, and global powers, institutions and establishments have tried and are still trying desperately to keep control. On a personal level, our ego structures are being dismantled too, particularly those built on an over-dominance of the masculine (patriarchal) energy. If you remember, ego structures are the identities and labels we give ourselves, which our mind creates to give us a sense of safety and security.

These identities also mean we take on specific roles, but when we lose a job, for example, we can no longer call ourselves a performer, an air steward, a manager, etc., so we feel we lose a part of ourselves, then we experience loss and grief. As you now understand, loss and grief are a painful process, mainly because human beings are creatures of habit and for the most part hate change!

Although I have mentioned the patriarchal system as that being governed by males, please don't misunderstand me—I am not casting blame on biological men and those who identify as the male gender. If you remember back to the first half of this book, you now understand that all people, regardless of biological sex, have a mix of both masculine and feminine energy within trying to seek balance. Any way in which your personal masculine and feminine energies are imbalanced through your own ego structures (Saturn) from beliefs, conditioning, upbringing, even your natal birth chart, are also being dismantled (Pluto) in some way. Biological women, for example, can predominantly live more from their masculine energy—in fact, I was one of those women before I created union within. For example, do you live solely from the mind, disregarding your intuition? Do you take action with will and force, not allowing room for surrender and non-doing? Quite often, these imbalances within will manifest as an external experience or we will see them play out in others; we project them outward, so to speak, so we can see them more clearly. Sadly, many people don't bother to reflect and take notice but seek to further cast blame, rejecting in others that which is also part of themselves. This creates an even bigger divide between the ego conscious self (what is consciously known) and the shadow aspect of one's being (what is unknown). The world as seen through our two physical eyes then looks separated and dualistic in nature—me versus you, us versus them, right or wrong, good or evil—but it's an illusion, the very paradox of earthly life. However, when we view the world through our all-seeing spiritual third eye, we seek to bridge the gap and create union within. A merging of our masculine and feminine energy, harmony between the right and left side of our brains, heart and mind working together and not against each other. We then live from a place of balance where we can be BOTH/AND, which is non-binary... not simply one or the other, regardless of sex.

The End of an Age

Technically, in astrology when two planetary bodies meet, they are marking the end of a cycle but also the start of a new one—just like at every monthly new moon when the Sun and Moon come together in the sky, marking the end of the current lunar cycle and beginning the next (the full moon represents the halfway point). The meeting between Pluto and Saturn on 20 January 2020 was actually the end of a cycle that started way back in 1982, and as you now know, with all endings come change, loss and grief. It's important, then, that we process this great change and what loss this may bring so we may step fully into the new beginning when it presents itself. Often with loss, we will spend too long looking back. Our grief holds us to the past, which as you now understand, hinders the ability to live fully in the present. When we come to see that all life and the universe is cyclical and that we are bound by patterns of a repeating nature, we become more accepting of the death and rebirth process. For example, a farmer works with such a cycle; after ripe crops have been harvested, they reap the benefits of their hard work by selling their produce. Then they must plough their fields in preparation for sowing the seeds once again for the season that follows. Although sowing the seed marks the start of the next farming cycle, the seeds take time to grow deep in the soil, and the farmers won't get to see the roots pushing through the earth and sprouting until the following spring.

All cycles follow this similar process of transformation—incubation, conception, birth, growth, blossoming, followed by decay and finally death—they just have different lengths. The lunar cycle is monthly, the solar cycle is yearly and the Pluto and Saturn cycle is approximately a 33-year process. So the new cycle that was seeded on the 20th January 2020 might not be physically visible until 2027, akin to its birthing and spring phase (due to its longer cycle). Therefore, it's almost like the universe is holding us in a dark tunnel, a void and space between one cycle ending and the next being born. Ask yourself this... Is the pause between breaths the end of the last or the start of the next? It's hard to tell, right? It's hard to tell at what point the end has taken place and the new has begun, and we are in this place now. That's not to say that nothing will happen for the next seven years; we only have to look at the magical and profound transformation that the female human body undergoes during pregnancy to see much is taking place, even if we can't initially see it. From the point of conception (which is unseen) to the actual birth of the baby (the physical manifestation), a tremendous metamorphic transformation takes place.

Therefore, humanity as a whole is currently experiencing a deep transformation, albeit unconsciously for many, but change is taking place within the hearts, minds and psyches of everyone on the planet right now. Unlike with a baby, we can't perceive or picture the new world that will be born in the future, and we don't have an ultrasound scan to check that everything is unfolding as it should. All we can do is hold hope, love and peace in our hearts, because the transformation needs to happen inside of us before it can physically manifest in the outer world.

If we look at all Pluto and Saturn conjunctions for the last century, you can see that they occurred at times of great upheaval and power struggles. 1982 saw the Falklands War between Argentina and the United Kingdom, 1947 saw the Cold War between Russia and Western countries, and in 1914

World War I began. The next Pluto and Saturn conjunction will take place in 2053 and I'll be 74 years old, which is a crazy thought, and we will be seeing how the end of the cycle seeded now in 2020 is playing out! So what you do now will create what will manifest in your world three decades from now; we really are creating the world for future generations. However, a Pluto and Saturn conjunction in Capricorn alone wasn't big enough to create the transformation that the universe requires for this millennium, and king of the gods himself—mighty Jupiter to the Romans and Zeus to the Greeks—also joined the party! It is an extremely rare occurrence to have all three of these planets in Capricorn; in fact the last time it happened was over 700 years ago in 1285 at the end of the last crusades. Jupiter in astrology is generally considered good luck and associated with the principles of prosperity, abundance, growth and expansion. As such, he rules higher learning, knowledge, religion and faith. However, Jupiter isn't judgemental and expands anything he touches. That means, like a quartz crystal, he can amplify positive and negative energy—or what we perceive as good and bad. Jupiter entered Capricorn in December of 2019 and orbits faster than Saturn and Pluto, taking eleven and a half years to complete one full cycle of the Sun and zodiac. So throughout the whole of 2020, Jupiter was catching up to his friends who were ahead of him. I find it mind blowing to see the coronavirus case numbers increased within the UK around the two periods where Jupiter (expansion) was exactly conjunct Pluto (death) in Capricorn on the 4th April and 12th November 2020.

Jupiter did conjunct Pluto on 30th June 2020 also but was in retrograde motion, which means that from the perspective of Earth it looked like the planet was travelling backwards. Planetary retrogrades are a normal occurrence and see the planets retrace their earlier steps, so they backtrack earlier degrees of the zodiac that they have already travelled. So sometimes when you experience similar themes that repeat in your life, if you have astrological awareness you can begin to see those circumstances as a chance for you to re-do something. To learn something that perhaps you missed the first time around.

There were many other significant astrological events in 2020 involving other planets and lesser-known asteroids and celestial bodies, but I am keeping this as simple as I can for the purposes of this book. I just wanted to highlight how the energy created by the Pluto and Saturn conjunction, along with Jupiter transiting both, created the perfect ingredients for what became our reality here on Earth. I truly believe that if it hadn't been the outbreak of the coronavirus, something else would have caused the circumstances ripe for a global purging of grief. Ironically, the somewhat hidden and smallest microbe possible has had the biggest global impact by creating 'the great pause of 2020'. I also find it highly interesting that the coronavirus seems to targets the lungs, the organs associated with the emotions of grief and sadness in Traditional Chinese Medicine.

The Grand Mutation
At the time of writing, the show-stopping finale to 2020 is yet to occur, but will be a much more favourable end to one of the most difficult years any of us have ever seen before in our lifetimes. Another monumental conjunction and meeting will take place between two planets... this time it's Saturn and Jupiter's turn. They will come so close they will look like one big bright star in our night sky. This meeting will take place on 21st December 2020, the winter solstice here in the northern hemisphere, when one of Earth's poles is maximally tilted away from the Sun. As a result, we see our shortest day and longest night, where we will have maximum amount of darkness and minimum amount of light; therefore, this day is one of the four shift points in Earth's seasonal cycle. Autumn ends and winter begins, and for the southern hemisphere, spring ends and summer begins. If you remember, a conjunction is where two planets seem to align in the sky and meet at the exact same degree of the zodiac, marking the ending of one cycle and the beginning of another. So the new

beginning seeded on this day will be extra potent due to the energy of the solstice.

However, it's not a farmer planting seeds in the soil or a female egg being fertilised by sperm; it's the two largest planetary bodies in our solar system, structure-forming Saturn and mighty giver Jupiter seeding the skies... the cosmic womb! Saturn and Jupiter come together in this way approximately every 20 years, however 2020 has been no ordinary year and this conjunction is no exception. It's an extremely rare occurrence known as a Grand Mutation and marks the start of not only a new Jupiter and Saturn 20-year cycle but also the beginning of a 200-year Air Era. This means we shift from their cycles, starting in the element of earth, to the element of air, and the lucky zodiac sign to birth their new 200-year cycle is Aquarius. The flavour of Aquarius energy is original, inventive, visionary, futuristic, revolutionary, freedom-seeking and even a little rebellious. Aquarius represents 'the people'—communities and groups coming together for the greater good—and in my opinion, is the zodiac sign most often misunderstood. Also known as the water-bearer, Aquarius, whose glyph looks like two parallel wavy water lines, and is depicted as the gods watering and nourishing the Earth, is often mistaken for a water sign. However it actually symbolises two lines of electricity running through the air, because Aquarius is ruled by planet Uranus, who in Greek Mythology was Ouranos, the God of the vast celestial heavens and sky. Uranus represents electricity, lightening, technology, the genius and sudden flashes of heavenly insight. The water-bearer's vase or container therefore is the structure and form that Capricorn energy brings (the sign that comes before Aquarius), and the water represents the nourishment of divine essence and spirit, the energy that comes from Pisces (the sign after it). So Aquarius is the link between the elements of earth and water. It is also the new age that humanity is currently entering.

The Birth of a New Age
If you are old enough, you may remember back to the much anticipated New Year of 1999 and all the hype regarding the

end of the world. People thought that planes were going to start dropping out the sky and that the Earth would suddenly stop rotating... fear-mongering and misinformation at its best! Then, again, on the 21st December 2012, news and social media was rife with doomsday and apocalyptic end of the world stories. Although I am no expert on the subject, I do know that the Maya Long Count Calendar, which is like an ancient astronomical clock, was the source of the prediction; however, I believe it was misinterpreted. It never predicted 'the end of the world', but the end of the world as we knew it... It predicted 'the end of an age'.

To be more precise, the end of the Piscean Age that began back at the time of Jesus—note that Pisces' glyph is two fishes swimming in opposite directions. Perhaps we were simply misinformed... after all, our timeline or Gregorian calendar is a manmade creation invented by Pope Gregory XIII in 1582. Although there is much debate between cosmologists and astrologists as to the exact start and end of such an age, which are cycles of approximately 2100 years, most agree that somewhere in this millennium we will indeed enter the Age of Aquarius, a time when a new civilisation will emerge, based on co-operation, peace and more humanitarian values where quantum leaps will be made in science, medicine, space travel and all things technological. As I previously mentioned, the twelve signs of the zodiac split the sky into 30-degree sections. Zero degrees is the first degree of each zodiac sign and 29 degrees the last, and the Jupiter and Saturn Grand Mutation is taking place at the very potent birthing point where all possibilities exist... the zero point! So even if we haven't officially begun the new age according to some calculations, we are most certainly about to enter it. Pluto, the slowest moving of the traditional planets, however, won't join his buddies in Aquarius until 19th November 2024, where he will remain for 20 years.

So, in summary, we are simultaneously being asked to be death doulas to an old world and midwives to help birth a new one. The new beginning being seeded in December of 2020 will see the hierarchal pyramid structures our societies have been built on (Saturn) re-energised in innovative and pioneering ways (Aquarius) that foster beliefs and faith (Jupiter) based on co-operation, equality and humanitarianism. But for the new to be born, the old age must also die, which was set into motion by the January 2020 conjunction of Pluto and Saturn— both of whom are, by the way, considered malefic planets in astrology, meaning they supposedly bring bad luck and misfortune. While you could look at 2020 with all its natural disasters, social upheaval, riots, civil unrest, political turmoil, economic recession, pandemic and other challenges and conclude that there is truth in such an assumption, I prefer to take the stance of unity as opposed to duality—the polarised thinking of something being good or bad. When you view things from a higher perspective and ultimately from truth, you see that all energy has a positive and negative charge; all planets therefore have light AND shadow qualities to them. Like the ancient Chinese Yin-Yang symbol, there is some positive always found in a negative situation. It's your perception that dictates if you see it.

I must be honest—I was highly apprehensive about including this chapter on astrology in a self-help book on anxiety, fear, loss and grief, but my spirit guides assured me that people would be ready to hear it. That humanity is ready to revolutionise the way they think and do things, to live in a more free, loving, inclusive society where our unique and individual differences are honoured not condemned. Some people will welcome this paradigm shift while others will resist, kicking and screaming; either way, change will always come. In true Aquarian style, this is no ordinary self-help book as it shares beliefs, ideas and techniques outside of the 'normal' sphere of thinking. It includes new concepts of self-governance and self-regulation that some will be unwilling to accept as a new way to live, but that's ok, everyone will grow and evolve in their own time when their consciousness is ready. Ironically, Uranus, the planet who breaks new ground and likes to do things differently, rules Aquarius and actually oversees astrology! Another confirmation to me that these words must be written.

The Great Spiritual Awakening
The good news is... more and more people are ready to do things differently because humanity has begun and continues to undergo a mass spiritual awakening. Many are experiencing shifts in their total being from an expansion of consciousness. Having faith is much more than following a particular religion or belief; it means trusting in something that you can't sometimes understand or physically see. It is trusting your own knowing and experience and not just blindly following what others believe or say, which brings me to the elusive realm of Neptune. To the Romans, he was god of waters and seas, and to the Ancient Greeks, he was Poseidon the 'earth-shaker', who was depicted with a horse and trident and believed to be responsible for earthquakes. Neptune is also another of the slowly moving outer plants who takes nearly 165 years to travel around the Sun, spending 15 years in each zodiac sign. Neptune rules the zodiac sign of Pisces, and actually moved into its home sign in February 2012 and will remain there until March 2025. The last time Neptune was home in Pisces was in 1862, and so not one person living on this planet has ever before experienced this energy until now. So just like Saturn has been super powered up in Capricorn, its home sign, Neptune in Pisces is extra happy and powerful there too.

Neptune represents formlessness, spirit and the ocean of divine consciousness, so rules over spirituality, mysticism, dreams, receptivity, visions, the psychic realms and altered states of reality. Pisces is a mutable water element whose flavour is inspiring, creative, imaginative and intuitive. Pisces energy has trouble defining its self; this is due to its ultra-sensitive and dissolving nature, which could be compared to a separate drop of water reuniting and merging with the ocean once more. The same could be said for our spark of individual consciousness, which is unified with the divine essence of all that is when one finds enlightenment. It's therefore no surprise to see the recent surge in the New Age spiritual movement and a revival of ancient mystical and spiritual practices spreading across the globe. However, now is the time to create your own faith based on your own truth, experience and innate wisdom, because Neptune in Pisces is opening us up, helping dissolve our limiting boundaries and beliefs so we can create our own unique connection with the divine. Neptune in Pisces is letting the light in; it's where we gain access to the divine source of creation while in body, reminding us that union with the great intelligence will always be possible. However, discernment is most definitely needed when you start opening up in this way, because Neptune in Pisces is evasive, elusive, nebulous and indecisive and so can be easily influenced by other energies, causing confusion and in some cases delusion. Always listen to your gut and intuition, and don't blindly follow someone that is seen as a spiritual 'guru', leader or religious teacher. Become your own authority. Also, water—just like the other elements—can be viewed from a dualistic perspective, so although purifying and soothing, it can also be overpowering and destructive, like a surging wave or tsunami that sweeps you away. So watch out for the negative or shadow side of Neptune in Pisces, which can bring illusions and escapism, a wanting to 'check out' from the harsh reality of earthly life, possibly leading to drugs, addiction, self-harm and other self-destructive behaviours.

Interestingly, both Pisces and its ruling planet Neptune both oversee the last section of the natal birth chart known as the 12th House, the House of shadow, self-undoing and isolation. Unlike Pluto and Scorpio who rule the 8th House which ask us to consciously delve into our psyche to transform, Neptune, Pisces and the 12th House is our unconscious capacity, so it's where we lose ourselves and experience dissolution. As such, the 12th House represents hospitals, jails, nursing homes, mental asylums and the end of life. I find it fascinating that when I was experiencing extreme dissociation, depersonalisation and derealisation after my spiritual trauma, Neptune in the sky was exactly conjunct with my birth Moon, which represents our subconscious, habitual patterns and reactions, our past and our ancestors. In fact, if I had more time, I would conduct research regarding mental illness and astrology transits, because I believe that the mental health pandemic which has swept our modern society even before the coronavirus erupted is partly due to this planetary energy being felt here on Earth. According to the World Health Organisation, 800,000 die from suicide every year. That's one person every 40 seconds. A recent report by the Samaritans in 2019 ([20]) showed that suicide rates in the UK were the highest they'd been since 2013... Just to note, that's one year after Neptune moved into Pisces. Data showed that the suicide rates of young females were at their highest rate on record and that there was also a significant rise in male suicides. Men were around three times more likely than women to take their own lives in the UK, which further highlights the need to stop the stigma around mental illness. This must include how emotions are perceived and managed by gender and sex. The conditioned gender-stereotypical belief that 'men or boys must not cry' and that 'women and girls are too emotional or sensitive' has done extreme damage to us as individuals and to us collectively as human beings. Certainly in Western countries there has been an over-reliance on physical health, neglecting the equally important emotional and mental health. I feel the suicide statistics yet to be collated will bring a sobering reminder of how each and every single one of us is fighting an inner battle to remain stable in a world that has become incredibly imbalanced.

In April 2020, Neptune reached 20 degrees of Pisces, which means we are now in the last ten degrees of the sign which features a more Scorpionic and Plutonian undertone (due to something called Decans in astrology). So until March 2025, the remaining four years Neptune is in Pisces, there will be an extra push from the universe to uncover what is secret and hidden in the psyche, a process which is uncomfortable, especially when we feel we are made to go there. So be prepared for things to seem initially worse before they get better. Sometimes things have to fall apart so they can be put back together from a more stable and balanced foundation. Remember, it is always darkest before the dawn, and Neptune is the light shining into our shadow. If we can see this as a final opportunity to purge and release any old outdated programming, beliefs, conditioning, unprocessed trauma, loss and grief, we will find more peace within where a renewed faith and personal rebirth arises. Human beings at this time are processing that which took many lifetimes in the past, so give yourself a big pat on the back! The great benefic Jupiter, who—if you remember—expands everything he touches, also enters Pisces in May 2021, so between then and December 2022, the above Pisces themes of heightened intuition, sensitivity, seeing what is hidden and endings will be even more amplified. Especially when Jupiter meets with Neptune at 23 degrees of Pisces in April 2022.

This final push of purging will be especially relevant when Pluto reaches the final degree of Capricorn for the first time in February 2023. Just like the zero degree is potent in offering new beginnings where all possibilities exist, the crucial and urgent 29th degree is potent for finishing up! This will bring a sense of urgency within the collective to do this deep soul-searching work whether they want to or not. Although Pluto does move into Aquarius for a short stint from March to June 2023, due to Pluto's retrogrades (remember, that's a change in direction from the perspective of Earth where the planet shifts from forward motion to travelling backwards) he will travel back to the 29th degree of Capricorn several times. Eventually, Pluto will finish his sixteen-year stay in Capricorn with a bang because he will make the mother of all retrogrades where he will station direct at 29'39 degrees on 12th October 2024. When a planet 'stations', it kind of comes to a stand-still, and as a consequence the energy builds and accumulates, which means it can be felt here on Earth much more intensely around these times, so mark these dates in your diaries! Then finally, on 20 November 2024, we say 'sayonara' to Pluto in Capricorn and welcome the planet into Aquarius. Then some four months later on 31

March 2025, Neptune also shifts signs, from Pisces to Aries, all of which are huge energetic shifts... The world will feel and look a whole lot different by then!

A Better You... A Better World
I haven't always looked up to the sky, but I have always looked inwards. From a young age, I guess I tried to find the meaning in things, and as for many, the answers seemed to elude me. I would often contemplate the meaning of life and ask myself the hundred million dollar question... 'Why am I here?' What all religions past and present have sought to understand and explain, I guess, but I never felt content to take another point of view as my own. I felt more comfortable to seek and find my own truth. However, I didn't realise I was on a quest of self-discovery, as my intention was only ever to be what I saw as healthy in mind and body, happy and fulfilled. From all the knowledge and experience I have gathered, I can't say that one therapy, one area of study or method of self-development was better than another. Reiki and meditation definitely created a strong foundation for me, but all disciplines played a significant part of a much larger process. Like pieces of a puzzle make a whole picture, it was astrology for me that seemed to just join all the pieces together.

Looking back, I always read my horoscope, more out of curiosity and for entertainment than anything, but it wasn't until the year 2000 that I saw an advert on the university intranet by a member of staff who was offering a birth chart reading for a tenner that sparked a real interest for me (eternally grateful to you, Hazel). I then started reading articles, Googling what things meant and studying my own birth chart in great detail and over time accumulated a whole book's worth of information. I'm by no means an expert astrologer, and the more I learn I feel the less I know, which would be highly frustrating for many but seems to please my fast and inquisitive mind. I feel I was divinely guided to study it and am so grateful to those astrologers who I listened to and learnt from, because it's what really got me through my biggest challenge of all, my Dark Night of the Soul and PTSD. Having astrological insight didn't stop my trauma and experiences, but it did give me understanding where I could logically see and conceptualise what I was so deeply feeling and experiencing. It also helped me to accept the impermanence of all things, which during difficult times is a relief, to know that nothing stays the same. I can't help but think of the old Persian adage written by the ancient Sufi poets... 'This too shall pass!' You see, astrology when used correctly is like a road map for your life, and for me, forewarned is forearmed. A bit like knowing what ingredients you've got before being expected to cook a meal means you can prepare and use the ingredients in the best combinations. Transit astrology, which is knowing where the planets are in the sky in real-time, shows if your own planetary placements in your birth chart are being activated or triggered. This helps you to know what type of energy is available to you in each passing moment and what lessons you may be facing, not to be restricted by the information but to assist you in making wiser choices. People watch the weather forecast, right?! If it shows heavy rain for the morning, you might choose to leave your gardening for the brighter afternoon. You can't stop the rain, that's the nature of life, but you can plan your day better. Knowing what cosmic weather is at play, to me, is no different really. However, what I found most rewarding was what I uncovered from understanding my own natal birth chart. All my deepest nuances, needs, desires, inner conflicts, confusions and dilemmas were not some fault or malfunction but could be explained by the energies that were present at the time of my birth. As such I came to fully accept myself exactly as I am. By accepting myself, I became more tolerant, patient and less judgemental of others, accepting them exactly as they are too.

I have spoken mostly of the longer generational planetary cycles that take effect over many years; however, what are known as the personal planets, namely the Sun, Moon, Mercury, Mars and Venus, move through the zodiac signs much faster, so change the energies available to us here on Earth more frequently. The Moon, for example, changes zodiac signs every two and a half days and reflects our feelings, inner rhythms and emotional reality, along with our subconscious habitual behaviours and patterns. Your moon energy is what you do once home and alone, how you self-soothe and comfort yourself, the part of your personality that perhaps only close family or friends get to see. Knowing your moon sign alone can help shed a huge light on your processing of grief because it rules how you process emotions in general. Maybe you get frustrated because you find it difficult to tap into your emotions, so perhaps your moon is in Capricorn or Aquarius? Or maybe like me you cry at TV adverts—the Moon was in a water sign at the time of my birth. Most people know what their Sun sign is—that's the horoscope you would read in the paper. People state 'I'm a Gemini', for instance, but what they are actually saying is, 'The Sun, our star and centre of our solar system, was in the sign of Gemini when I was born.' The Sun represents your identity, your star quality, core essence and vitality. It plays a significant factor in your fundamental personality, which further creates your conscious self and ego structures. However, there are another nine traditional planets that represent a different part of you and your personality somewhere in the sky in one of the twelve signs of the zodiac and are not necessarily in the same sign as your sun. The natal birth chart not only shows what zodiac signs all the planets fell in at the time of your birth, but it is also further split into different areas or Houses. These represent different themes that you experience as you journey through life, different sectors such as family, communication, career, relationships, etc. So although the mega-purge and death of old structures (the January 2020 Pluto and Saturn conjunction) took place in Capricorn, that will be in a different area of everyone's chart and thus manifesting in a different area of your life. It took place in my 4th House, of family and roots, which explains why I was asked to heal and release ancestral wounding from this and past lives. I obviously didn't do a good enough job at transforming my loss and grief in previous incarnations. Your unique natal birth chart is like a personal star map which not only takes you on an outer journey to the sky above you but more importantly takes you on a journey home, inward to your inner cosmos.

Although I had studied the concept of astrology on a mental level for almost fifteen years, it wasn't until my PTSD in 2016 and experiencing my own great pause in grief that my connection to the cosmos profoundly deepened. My ability as an Earth Empath grew and began to include other planets too, and I began to sense planetary energies very viscerally in my own physical body. It was overwhelming at first, but over time I managed to understand what certain physical sensations meant and what planets they were connected to. I also came to realise that much of my health anxiety over the years had actually been due to these sometimes strange yet very real and somatic sensations I would have. It sounds very farfetched, I know, but our physical bodies really are instruments that can detect vibration and frequency changes; some are just more sensitive to them than others. The planetary energies would often manifest themselves in my dreams too, in human form to speak with me directly, which I know sounds absolutely bat-shit crazy, but it's the truth and I know I am not crazy. Like many people who first discover astrology, I couldn't help but feel a sense of fate at play initially, which if I am honest, I was completely uncomfortable with. At first I felt I was machine-like and almost being controlled, at the mercy of the planetary energies and influences with no say in my life, which is obviously untrue. Astrology shows trends, possibilities and what is available energetically within and also around us, but of course what you do with those possibilities and how you navigate your life through the decisions you make is totally up to you. We will always have free will and can work with the universe in a symbiotic way, but it is a choice. Carl Jung was the man responsible for the concept of 'synchronicity', which postulates that events are 'meaningful coincidences' if they occur with no causal relationship yet seem to be meaningfully related. Jung actually called astrology 'the science of antiquity' and told Sigmund Freud in a letter in 1911 'my evenings are largely taken up with astrology. I make horoscopic calculations in order to find a clue to the core of psychological truth. Some remarkable things have turned up which will certainly appear incredible to you.' [21] I share this information with you now not to sell or to preach but to simply highlight how astrology helped me. Even if you never go on to study and understand your own birth chart, I hope that you can at least begin to see the bigger picture of 2020... the year the world paused.

We are part of something vast and meaningful, in some ways beyond human comprehension, and astrology has helped me to connect to the great mystery that is the cosmos in a more conscious and tangible way. My lifelong journey inward to find myself has so far taught me that my purpose is to make the unseen seen, to make what is hidden visible and to demystify the mysterious. Through understanding myself, I have had the honour and privilege of helping others understand themselves. Had I not faced my own fears, I wouldn't have been able to help others face theirs, especially the most fundamental fear of all... death. Although I unconsciously helped both my nans transform state from the physical to the ethereal, it wasn't until February 2019 that I willingly and knowingly helped my Grampy pass over, only one year before I would be called to start assisting the mass passing of souls who have and continue to leave our earthly plane in 2020. And to those who have lost a loved one during this time, please know that they were not alone. Not only were the brave doctors and nurses physically beside them, but also the hundreds of people around the world like myself who at this time are stepping up and becoming who they are meant to be, helping humanity energetically at a very dark hour.

Any self-development work at its root is true spirituality, which is finding your true self! It isn't all 'love and light' but involves bravery and commitment, an unlearning of everything you have been conditioned to believe is true. A letting go of all the things you think you are or are not. All the things other people have told you you are or are not. A throwing off of the shackles that have kept you stuck, contained and confined. We live on one planet, but each of us lives in our own world created by our experiences, our thoughts, feelings, beliefs, upbringing, conditioning, family and culture. But beyond that, underneath all the layers, the ego and all the names, labels and concepts, there is a part of each of us that is completely unaffected by physical life. Many religions and ancient esoteric teachings have tried to rationalise and conceptualise such an idea, and as a result there have been many different names and terms used to explain such a concept, all from their very own specific perspective. Most people have heard of the terms spirit and soul, but there are many other words used to describe our non-physical elusive self. Terms such as higher-self, macro-self, spiritual-self, etheric-self, transcended-self, divine-self, metaphysical-self, astral body, aura, monad, spark, divine masculine, divine feminine, etc.

Then there are the many words used to describe the non-physical life force that permeates all living beings, such as: chi, ki, prana, energy, mana, kama, shakti, vibe, essence, spark, vital energy, kundalini, force, power, subtle energy, etc. While it wouldn't serve the purpose of this book to give an explanation of each, their similarities and subtle differences, I will share my most fundamental knowing. To our mind, time exists with a definitive end, but to our spirit, time is eternal. Your soul and its evolution is attached to karma, which influences your time and place of birth therefore your culture, conditioning, programming, habits, trauma, ancestral wounding, traits and states of being—all of which create your unique reality in this and every life you have ever lived and will live. Your spirit, however, is infinite and changeless, so therefore will live on, not only in the hearts and minds of those you love but in time and space.

Energy cannot die or be destroyed; it can only transform state. Your spirit is pure and perfect, always has and always will be.

I understand that all the information contained within this book won't appeal to all readers, and of course there are many roads that lead to the same destination. Mastering yourself is about finding what works for you. There are numerous self-development methods, therapies, belief systems and ways of living that may be more suited to you, but I hope you now feel inspired to seek and find your own answers if you couldn't find them within this book. It is my hope that by reading *Mastering Your Crown*, you not only learn to cope better throughout this pandemic, but you come out victorious. Closer to knowing yourself more fully, knowing your own strength, your own worth, your own uniqueness and in better health, more whole in mind, body and energy.

Just as one pebble cast into a lake creates ripples that reach out far and wide, mastering yourself will inspire those around you too, because a better you will also create a better world.

So what are you waiting for? Go get your crown!

REFERENCES

($_1$) Olff, M. (2017). *Sex and gender differences in posttraumatic stress disorder: an update.* European Journal of Psychotraumatology, Vol 8, Sup 4.

($_2$) McEwen, B, S. (2005). *Stressed or Stressed out: What's the Difference?* Journal of Psychiatry Neuroscience, 30 (05): 315-318.

($_3$) Aron, E. N., Aron, A. & Jagiellowicz, J. (2012). *Sensory Processing Sensitivity: A review in the Light of the Evolution of Biological Responsivity.* Personality & Social Psychology Review XX (X), p1-21.

($_4$) Lepletier, A., Hun, M. L, Hammett, M. V., Wong, K., Naeem, H., Hedger, M., & Chidgey, A. P. (2019). *Interplay between Follistatin, Activin A, and BMP4 Signaling Regulates Postnatal Thymic Epithelial Progenitor Cell Differentiation during Aging.* Cell Reports, 27(13), 3887-3901.

($_5$) Nasseri, F. & Eftekhari, F. (2010). *Clinical and Radiological Review of the Normal and Abnormal Thymus: Pearls and Pitfalls.* RadioGraphics, Volume. 30; No. 2, 413-428.

($_6$) Bretheron, B., Atkinson, L., Murray, A., Clancy, J. & Deuchars, J. (2019). *Effects of transcutaneous vagus nerve stimulation in individuals aged 55 years or above; potential benefits of stimulation.* Aging, Vol, 11, No 14.

($_7$) Stefanov, M., Potroz, P., Jungdae, K., Jake, L., Richard, Cha, & Min-Ho, Nam. (2013). *The Primo Vascular System as a New Anatomical System.* Journal of Acupuncture and Meridian Studies, 6 (6); 331338).

($_8$) Paul MacLean (1990). *The Triune Brain in Evolution. Role of Paleocerebral Functions.* Plenum, New York, xxiv, p672.

($_9$) Tully, R. B., Coutois, H., Hoffman. Y. & Pmarede, D. (2014). *The Laniakea supercluster of galaxies.* Nature, Volume 513, number 7516, p71.

($_{10}$) HeartMath Institute (2015). *Science of the Heart; Exploring the Role of the Heart in Human Performance, Volume 2.* An Overview of Research Conducted by HeartMath Institute.

(11) https://cristales.fundaciondescubre.es/?page_id=1769

(12) Reznikov, N., Bilton, M., Lari, L., Stevens, M. & Kroger, R. (2018). *Fractal-like hierarchical organisation of bone begins at the nanoscale.* Science, 4 May, Volume 360, Issue 6388, p2189.

(13) Cook, W. & Cook, W. (2012). *Universal Truths; Unlocking the Secrets to Energy Healing.* Wanda Cook Publishing.

(14) https://www.worldometers.info/coronavirus/

(15) Cowen, A. S. & Keltner, D. (2017). *Self-report captures 27 distinct categories of emotion bridged by continuous gradients.* PNAS Early Edition, Feb, p1-10.

(16) Brannan, D., Davis, A. & Biswas-Diener, R. (2016). *The Science of Forgiveness: Examining the Influence of Forgiveness on Mental Health.* Encyclopaedia of Mental Health, Volume 2, p253-256.

(17) Hirshkowitz, M. et al. (2015). *National Sleep Foundation's sleep time duration recommendations; methodology and results summary.* Sleep Health, Marc; 1; (40-43).

(18) Porkka-Heiskanen, T., Alanko, L., Kalinchuk, A. & Stenburg, D. (2002). *Sleep and Adenosine. Sleep Medicine Reviews,* Volume 6, issue 4, July, p321-332.

(19) Radin, D., Hayssen, G., Emoto, M., & Kizu, T. (2006). *Double-Blind Test of the Effects of Distant Intention of Water Crystal Formation.* Explore, Sept/Oct, Volume 2, No. 5, p408-411.

(20) Samaritans. (2019). *Suicide Statistics Report; Latest statistics for the UK and Republic of Ireland, December 2019.*

(21) Jung, C. G. (2018). *Jung on Astrology; Selected and Introduced by Safron Rossi and Keiron Le Grice.* Routledge.

APPENDIX A

Mental Health Resources

Anxiety UK
A charity providing support if you have been diagnosed with an anxiety condition.
Phone: 03444 775 774
Website: www.anxietyuk.org.uk

Cruse Bereavement Care
A charity which provides free care and bereavement counselling to people suffering from grief.
Phone: 0808 808 1677
Website: www.cruse.org.uk

Mental Health Foundation
A mental health charity focused on prevention.
Website: www.mentalhealth.org.uk

Mind
A mental health charity in England and Wales.
Phone: 0300 123 3393
Website: www.mind.org.uk

No Panic
A charity offering support for sufferers of panic attacks and obsessive compulsive disorder (OCD).
Phone: 0844 967 4848
Website: www.nopanic.org.uk

Papyrus UK
A national charity offering support to under-35s who are experiencing thoughts of suicide, as well as people concerned about someone else.
Phone: 0800 068 4141
Website: www.papyrus-uk.org

Rethink Mental Illness
Advice and information service.
Phone: 0300 5000 927
Website: www.rethink.org

Samaritans
Confidential support for people experiencing feelings of distress and despair.
Phone: 116 123
Website: www.samaritans.org.uk

Shout Crisis Text Line 85258
A free, confidential, 24/7 text messaging support service for anyone who is struggling to cope.
Text: 85258
Website: www.giveusashout.org

APPENDIX B

ABOUT THE AUTHOR

Emma Gholamhossein is a Health & Well-being Advisor, Exercise Specialist, Energy Therapist, Reiki Master Teacher, Psychic Healer, Angel Communicator and Cosmic Guide.

Emma has over 20 years' experience in the well-being, exercise and fitness industry, having taught every level of clientele from young children to more specialist groups, such as those with medical conditions and elite sportsmen and sportswomen. Emma's love of fitness has seen her teaching a range of specialist activities, including: aerobics, Pilates, power chi yoga, Trigger Point Pilates, TRX, spinning, kettlebells and boxercise to name just a few! Emma has a Bachelor of Science Degree (BSc) in Sports Coaching and a Master of Science Degree (MSc) in Physical Activity & Health. Emma is also a member of the Chartered Institute for the Management of Sport and Physical Activity (CIMSPA) and holds Senior Activity and Health Practitioner status.

Emma has over 10 years' experience as an Energy Therapist and is a Reiki Master Practitioner and Teacher, a Crystal Therapist, Metatronia Master Healer and a Thought Field Therapist. Emma is a member of the Federation of Holistic Therapists (FHT) as a Complementary and Sports Member and a Member of the Complementary Health Care Register Accredited by the Professional Standards Authority.

Emma is a psychic healer and can see a person's aura, energy body and inside the physical body, which greatly assists her in getting to the root cause of any issues, whether physical, mental, emotional or spiritual. This ability also allows Emma to communicate with the Angelic Realm, plus other energy beings, and also to sense planetary energies, thus allowing Emma to be a Cosmic Guide, Spiritual Coach and Earth-Keeper.

To learn more about Emma's services, please visit her website www.emmagholamhossein.com or visit her Facebook page 'Emma Gholamhossein' for regular interactives and inspirations.

APPENDIX C

ABOUT MASTERING ME

Emma is the founder of 'Mastering Me', where she teaches others how to master their mind, body and subtle energies. 'Mastering Me' assists others to reclaim their own power, helping them take responsibility to create a happier, healthier and more abundant life where they become the master of themselves.

Mastering Me Subscription Group

Emma runs a Mastering Me Subscription Group via Facebook where she helps others shift their energy and perspective, breaking free from old habits and beliefs. You will delve deeper into your own unique journey and learn new self-development methods where you become more whole, happy and content. It is your chance to work directly with Emma, and you also have the convenience of tuning in at a time that suits you and your lifestyle.

Mastering Me Body Subscription Group

Emma also runs a Mastering Me Body Subscription Group via Facebook where she helps others learn how to love, honour and heal their physical body. Over time you will discover that tension, stress and trauma held within your body melts away, tightness and restrictions release, muscles lengthen, pain eases and posture improves. Over time you will feel more embodied and confident in your own skin. Emma has created the Mastering Me Body Class using all her knowledge, experience and expertise as an Exercise Specialist and body worker. You will also have the convenience of tuning in at a time that suits you and your lifestyle

FREE Download
Mastering My Crown; Self Discovery Journal

Scan the following QR Code or visit
www.emmagholamhossein.com
to download the free Self Discovery Journal
that accompanies this book.

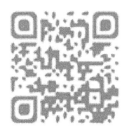

Lightning Source UK Ltd.
Milton Keynes UK
UKHW020659150921
390602UK00010B/222